Diagnostic
Procedures

Diagnostic Procedures
A Reference for Health Practitioners and a Guide for Patient Counseling

Barbara Skydell, R.N., M.S.

Former Instructor in Staff Development,
Columbia-Presbyterian Medical Center,
New York, New York

Anne S. Crowder, R.N., M.A.

Assistant Director of Nursing Education,
Burke Rehabilitation Center,
White Plains, New York

Little, Brown and Company
Boston

Published November 1975

Copyright © 1975 by Barbara Skydell and
Anne S. Crowder

First Edition
Second Printing

Library of Congress catalog card No. 75-30303

ISBN 0-316-79733-2

Printed in the United States of America

How often has the health professional been told that a diagnostic procedure must be rescheduled because the patient was uncooperative? How often has the patient been met with hostile, angry reactions from the staff because he could not or would not follow directions? How many times have patients stated, "If only I had known what to expect!" This manual is addressed to the patient's need and right to know why a procedure is being performed, what it will feel like, and what will be expected of him. It is therefore directed to the professionals who daily prepare patients for diagnostic procedures. It is specifically geared to provide information on which to draw in preparing the individual patient. Our intent is that the book will be used as a starting point for creative teaching of the patient and his family.

The procedures covered in the manual are not all-inclusive. We have selected those that are most commonly performed and for which the health professional most often prepares patients. We have also included many procedures which, although not widely performed, represent major refinements of or alternatives to current diagnostic techniques.

This book was originally written as a resource manual for the surgical nursing staff at Columbia-Presbyterian Medical Center. Because of the encouragement of our colleagues and the expressed need for just such a manual, it has been rewritten, expanded, and generalized so that it may be of use in any health care setting. Regretfully we have used the universal pronoun *he* when referring to the patient and *she* when speaking of the practitioner. This has been done for the sake of brevity only.

In preparing this manual we have made use of the abundance of material pertaining to the subjects; we have observed all the procedures; and, most important, we have consulted with patients who have experienced these procedures and the physicians who perform them. Furthermore, we have applied the principles and information included in this manual in our own activities and have found, without exception, that this has been effective and appreciated.

This manual is not intended to be a definitive reference on either a procedure or its diagnostic implications. Rather, it is offered as an immediate source of information for patient instruction and family inquiries. Where further in-depth material is required or desired, reference may be made to the bibliographies of nursing and medical publications specific to the subject.

The material made available to prepare a patient for any procedure must take into consideration that he is an individual interacting in many spheres. To detail all the ramifications of such preparation for each test would be repetitious and lacking in value. However, this aspect of the total preparation is crucial to the patient's experience of the procedure and often to its successful completion. Effort must be expended on choosing and employing appropriate communication tools. To enable the health professional more easily and effectively to include this sensitive area of care in planning patient teaching, a section on assessing learning needs is included. The material presented is intended to give structure to the health worker's thinking by providing avenues for exploration of the individual patient's receptivity to instruction.

From the suggestions and information provided, we hope the health professional will be able to integrate knowledge of the individual patient, theory, and professional judgment to extract and apply what is most pertinent and appropriate for each person and situation.

Many people have been of assistance in the preparation of this manuscript, far more than we can name here. We would like to express our appreciation and gratitude to all of them, especially for sharing and supporting the concept underlying this book, the patient's right to know. Particular thanks are extended to the following, who gave most freely and generously of their time, intellect, and patience: Richard A. Baker, M.D., William Casserella, M.D., D. Jackson Coleman, M.D., David Follett, M.D., Norman Joffe, M.D., Philip M. Johnson, M.D., Donald L. King, M.D., Arthur Smith, M.D., and the late Ernest H. Wood, M.D. To Lois Miles, R.N., go our special thanks for her involvement in the preparation of the material for the initial manual. We are especially indebted to Ruth Korn, R.N., for the preliminary research on the ophthalmology procedures. We offer our special appreciation to our parents, Harry and Rebecca Skydell and Richard and Helen Crowder, for a lifetime of continuous support and encouragement. And finally, to Josephine Fogarty we extend our thanks and gratitude for her patience and skill in deciphering, editing, and typing the manuscript.

B. S.
A. S. C.

Contents

Overview

An Approach to Communication

Will it hurt? What must I do? What if I have to go to the bathroom in the middle of the test? How can I be sure I won't disgrace myself in some way? Why are they repeating this test? Do I have cancer? Why can't I keep my dentures in? Why can't I wear my religious medal? Why do I have to wait so long? Have they forgotten about me? Why are they taking my blood pressure so often? Doesn't anybody care that I'm hungry?

These are some of the often unspoken concerns of patients undergoing diagnostic procedures. All too often preparation includes instituting the necessary dietary alterations and administering the appropriate premedications while the questions, fears, and concerns of the patient remain unanswered and untended. Often constraint of time is the reason; sometimes the health professional does not possess the necessary information regarding a particular procedure; and occasionally the health practitioner may not even be aware that such concerns and fears exist.

Preparation for diagnostic procedures must be individual and based on what the patient wants or needs to know in addition to what is required for the specific test. Some patients need to know all the whys and wherefores in order to maintain some semblance of control in an unfamiliar setting; others prefer a brief explanation; and still others express a desire to remain in ignorance. Preparation, then, also includes the manner in which one approaches, evaluates, and implements appropriate teaching to meet these individual needs.

Evaluation and determination of patient needs require specific knowledge and skills, many of which lie in the nebulous area of communication. Communication is an interchange involving not only talking to someone but also listening to what is being said, how it is being said, and evaluating the circumstances in which the interchange is taking place. Monitoring all the activity of both participants in the interchange requires objectivity, self-awareness, knowledge, and skill on the part of the professional person involved.

In order to appraise and achieve effective communication, it is helpful to consider some of the barriers which may impede or distort its intent or content.

Language is a major area to consider. Do you and your patient "speak the same language"? If your patient is from another country, command of a second language may be limited. Fear may further diminish his ability to deal with it. Equally, variations within a common language may be so disparate as to be almost incomprehensible. Whenever any disparity exists, the difference must be reconciled so that communication may be established, either verbally or nonverbally.

Preoccupation is a frequent barrier to communication. The patient is often concerned with matters not directly related to what is being communicated to him regarding the procedure. That which is occupying his mind may take many forms — severity of his illness, his physical condition, unattended children at home, absence from work, financial concerns, and so forth. Similarly, the health practitioner may be concerned with matters equally unrelated to the teaching process. Unless the preoccupation is recognized and dealt with, it may block further efforts to prepare the patient for the procedure.

Another problem is that which occurs when a patient thinks the staff is too busy to be bothered. Because of this assumption, the patient may suffer unnecessary fear or anxiety. Erroneous assumptions are made by the staff as well. How can there be any problems or questions?; the patient is "good" and never "bothers" anyone. Each then becomes the victim of the other's assumption, and communication is never established.

The perceptual framework of an individual plays a significant role in determining the way in which communication takes place. Differences in age, sex, ethnicity, and socioeconomic background between the patient and those caring for him are important influences. A negative response from either to the other's perceptual framework may compromise the potential for effective teaching and learning. The behavior and perceptions of an adolescent will differ from those of someone in the middle years. The norms and mores of one ethnic group will differ in some ways from those of another. A male nurse who prepares a female patient for a procedure may have difficulty establishing rapport if the woman is not accustomed to perceiving the man in that role. Differences in class may influence the manner in which the practitioner's status, and therefore authority, is viewed. Previous experience with illness may be crucial in determining how effective communication will be. If the illness and its treatment have been unpleasant, painful, or frightening, the patient will face his next encounter with the health care system, even for an unrelated cause, with great trepidation which may or may not be openly or directly expressed.

The informal means of communication within a hospital present unique problems. Words overheard at rounds, another patient's horror story of what he underwent during the same test, or the fearsome accounts of visitors may negatively affect the quality of the communication in the teaching-learning process. When this occurs, it will be necessary to go back, listen, explore the fears aroused, and reiterate the information that will allow the patient to prepare himself for the procedure without undue anxiety.

How does one move from recognition of these factors to actual implementation? Awareness allows the possibility of action. As professionals we have the responsibility to be aware of our own behavior as well as that of our patients and how each may affect the other. Begin by concentrating on what the patient is saying and doing. Listen carefully, be alert to nonverbal communication, and use the information gained from previous encounters.

With the information collected, one is in a position to make choices. How much information should be given? How should it be presented so that it is meaningful? What the patient wants to know or his command of the language may influence the choice of teaching tool, e.g., written versus verbal explanation, use of visual aids, or a tour of the radiology department. For example, preoccupation may necessitate dealing with the patient's primary concern first. It usually indicates providing information repetitively in small amounts or presenting the same information using varying methods as a means of reinforcement. Evaluation of the patient should dictate the choice of method and the amount of material to be presented.

Whatever method is chosen, feedback is necessary to allow for evaluation of the effectiveness of the teaching. Feedback means determining whether what has been taught to the patient is what the patient has learned. Feedback may be obtained directly, as by asking the patient to review what he has been taught, or indirectly through observation: the questions asked, facial expression, posture, activity, irritated response to information, apparent disinterest, or expressed concern about taking up too much time. Positive or negative feedback will then guide the instruction, whether the next step be reinforcement, more information, simpler words, pictures or diagrams, or a change in tone of voice or of implied attitude.

Regardless of the manner in which preparation is accomplished, the objective is to ensure congruency between what has been learned and the actuality of the event. Patients who know what to expect before, during, and after an unfamiliar procedure tolerate it with greater equanimity and with fewer deleterious physical and emotional effects.

Bibliography

Allen, E. M. Information viewed most helpful to patients undergoing three selected diagnostic procedures. *A.N.A. Clin. Conf.* p. 206, 1969.

Francis, G. M., and Munjas, B. *Promoting Psychological Comfort.* Dubuque, Iowa: Brown, 1968.

Janis, I. L. *Psychological Stress: Psychoanalytical and Behavioral Studies of Surgical Patients.* New York: Wiley, 1958.

Johnson, J. E., Morrissey, J. F., and Leventhal, H. Psychological preparation for an endoscopic examination. *Gastrointest. Endosc.* 19:180, 1973.

Redman, B. K. *The Process of Patient Teaching in Nursing* (2d ed.). St. Louis: Mosby, 1972.

Skipper, J. K., and Leonard, R. C. (Eds.). *Social Interaction and Patient Care.* Philadelphia: Lippincott, 1965.

Format and Commonalities

Each procedure in the manual follows a similar format. It includes purpose, time, location, personnel, equipment, technique, preparation, patient sensations, and aftercare. In an attempt to present information in the most meaningful way, the order of presentation varies with the procedure being described. When the same information is necessary in more than one procedure, the reader will be referred to the appropriate section.

The sections in each chapter are sequentially ordered. Reading the entire chapter will in some cases, notably ophthalmology, gastroenterology, and neurology, enhance the significance of the individual procedures. The reader is encouraged to read each procedure through entirely rather than search for a single piece of information under any one heading. Any particular item when taken out of context may serve to confuse rather than clarify.

A number of factors are common to successful completion of many of the procedures in this manual. To avoid repetition, they are omitted from the body of the text. Since many of them are common or obvious, these very qualities may cause them to be overlooked in the effort to implement the necessary specific preparations for a study. For these reasons they have been singled out for review and discussion here. Also included is an explanation of some of the terms used in the presentation of the procedures.

A. TIME
Questions concerning the scheduled time and usual duration of a procedure are frequently asked by patients. Whenever possible this information should be given with the caveat that many factors may affect its accuracy. Anyone who has experienced a diagnostic procedure, even one as simple as a chest x-ray, knows that waiting time far too often can exceed the time necessary to carry out the procedure. The patient must be forewarned of this possibility and advised to bring some diversional activity such as a book. Usually there is only a minimal wait when a major diagnostic procedure has been specifically scheduled.

Time as defined throughout the book refers only to the approximate length of the procedure. When preparing an inpatient, additional information should be given about time spent in waiting for transportation service, and in transit to and from the procedure. These factors often add considerably to the time a patient must spend away from the unit and cause him subjectively to experience the procedure as longer than it is. This perception may well add to his fatigue and may cause him to feel any side-effects of the procedure more acutely.

As many of the procedures may be lengthy, the patient should void before leaving the unit. Accommodating the patient's desire to void may be logistically difficult during a procedure.

B. PATIENT ATTIRE
What the patient is required to wear will vary with the situation. Most often hospitals require the patient to wear the traditional x-ray gown, while others in some instances permit the patient to wear his own clothing, be it pajamas or street clothes. When personal garb is permitted, the nature of the procedure and the positions the patient will be asked to assume should dictate the appropriate attire. For example, mammography requires that the breasts be exposed. A gown, pajama top, or blouse that can be removed easily would probably be most comfortable and convenient.

Particularly for radiological procedures, the patient should wear a robe and slippers if an inpatient, or carry a sweater if an outpatient. Radiology departments are notoriously cold.

C. CONSENT
Many diagnostic procedures require the patient's legally witnessed signature on a standard consent form. The policy of the individual institution will dictate the procedures for which this is necessary. To prevent frantic last-minute efforts to obtain consent and avoid possible cancellation and re-scheduling of the procedure with their inevitable physical, emotional, and financial costs incurred by the patient, the staff should know which procedures require a consent.

D. DIET
When a patient must be kept NPO for a particular procedure, we have merely stated this fact without specifying the exact number of hours involved. Dietary limitations and duration of fasting vary between institutions. Staff members should become familiar with their own protocols so that they can knowledgeably inform their patients. When a patient returns from a diagnostic procedure for which he has been kept fasting, he should be fed immediately if the examination has been completed. A missed breakfast may be perceived as lack of concern.

E. MEDICATIONS

Any patient being treated with medications where latitude as to time of administration is limited, e.g., insulin or quinidine, requires particular attention if fasting is necessary for a procedure. The patient's physician should be consulted as to which medications must be taken regardless of the fasting state.

Diuretics are an important class of drugs to consider. If the patient is to undergo a lengthy examination or the waiting time is likely to be long, it may be wise to withhold the diuretic, particularly a rapid-acting one such as furosemide, thereby saving the patient possible embarrassment or prolonged agony while undergoing the study.

The radiology department should be specifically informed by the patient or the hospital staff if the patient is a diabetic, and whether or not he has taken his insulin. Waiting time can thus be minimized and the patient's regimen not unduly altered.

F. PREMEDICATION

Specific premedications are rarely mentioned in the text, as the drugs or combination of drugs used varies considerably.

G. PERSONNEL

The staff members listed in this category are those usually involved in the procedure. This may vary from hospital to hospital. For some procedures we have stated that a radiologist performs the study. However, another specialist in a field related to the study may be the examiner, e.g., an orthopedic surgeon may perform anthrography.

Teaching hospitals often have students and other staff members present. Whenever possible, the situation most likely to pertain should be described to the patient. To arrive for a procedure expecting two or three people and to find instead a crowd of onlookers can be most disconcerting. It may to some extent reverse the careful preparation done and thereby impair the patient's ability to cooperate during the procedure.

H. RADIATION HAZARDS

As consumers of health care become more knowledgeable about matters pertaining to health, they are beginning to actively question some medical practices. One such practice on which much public attention has been focused is unnecessary exposure to radiation.

Patients scheduled for a radiological procedure should understand that before it is scheduled, the potential diagnostic yield is weighed against the hazards involved. Also, lead shields are used to protect the gonads in all radiological procedures except those such as intravenous pyelography in which gonadal exposure is inevitable.

Fluoroscopy is a major source of radiation. Diminution of this hazard has been accomplished by the development of image intensification, which decreases patient exposure time. When a procedure utilizing fluoroscopy is done, the patient should be informed that he is not being continuously exposed. The fluoroscope, though on repeatedly, is in operation for only a few seconds at a time. Staff involved with fluoroscopic examinations wear lead aprons. The patient should understand that the protective aprons are worn because the staff is continuously exposed to radiation on a daily basis, while the patient is not.

Finally, new diagnostic procedures are continually being developed to provide needed information at less risk to the patient. Radionuclide scanning procedures are relatively noninvasive and for the most part expose the patient to far lower amounts of radiation. Workers in this field are rapidly expanding the number of short-acting radiopharmaceuticals. Ultrasonography is another rapidly developing tool which does not utilize radiation at all. While many situations still require a more extensive, invasive radiological study, their number is being markedly reduced by these two relatively new diagnostic tools. In time they may obviate the need for many radiological studies.

I. EQUIPMENT

This category lists only the major or unusual items involved in performance of the procedure. Where appropriate, a photograph or a description of appearance and action has been provided.

J. PATIENT SENSATIONS

Under this category we have included the sensations experienced by the patient during preparation, throughout the actual procedure, and afterward. For clarity, some sensations are described in other sections of the procedure.

General Reading

Beranbaum, S. L., and Meyers, P. H. *Special Procedures in Roentgen Diagnosis.* Springfield, Ill.: Thomas, 1964.

Brunner, L. S., et al. (Eds.). *Textbook of Medical Surgical Nursing* (2d ed.). Philadelphia: Lippincott, 1970.

Chesney, D. N., and Chesney, M. O. *Care of the Patient in Diagnostic Radiography* (3d ed.). Philadelphia: Davis, 1970.

Jones, M. D. *Basic Diagnostic Radiology.* St. Louis: Mosby, 1969.

Meschan, I. *Analysis of Roentgen Signs in General Radiology.* Philadelphia: Saunders, 1973.

Paul, L. W., and Juhl, J. H. *The Essentials of Roentgen Interpretation* (3d ed.). New York: Harper & Row, 1972.

Potchen, E. J., Koehler, P. R., and David, D. O. *Principles of Diagnostic Radiology.* New York: McGraw-Hill, 1971.

Smith, D. W., and Gips, C. D. *Care of the Adult Patient* (2d ed.). Philadelphia: Lippincott, 1966.

Sutton, D. (Ed.). *A Textbook of Radiology.* Baltimore: Williams & Wilkins, 1969.

Thompson, T. T. *Primer of Clinical Radiology.* Boston: Little, Brown, 1973.

Weigen, J. F., and Thomas, S. F. *Complications of Diagnostic Radiology.* Springfield, Ill.: Thomas, 1973.

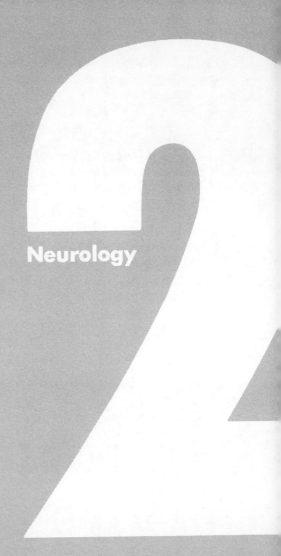

Neurology

Lumbar Puncture (Spinal Tap)

PURPOSE   Withdrawal of cerebrospinal fluid (CSF) by insertion of a thin hollow needle between the lower lumbar vertebrae into the subarachnoid space.

The procedure provides visual and laboratory information about the status of the brain and spinal cord such as elevated pressure, bleeding, spinal cord compression, and infection. Lumbar puncture may also be done for the administration of an anesthetic or medication or as part of another procedure, such as myelography, pneumoencephalography, or radioisotope cisternography.

TIME   Ten to 30 minutes. Placement of the needle may require more time if the patient is obese or has any spinal abnormalities such as kyphoscoliosis or osteoarthritis. Procedure time may also be extended if the CSF drips out slowly.

LOCATION   Patient's room or treatment room.

PERSONNEL   Physician and assistant.

EQUIPMENT   A 3 1/2-inch hollow needle with stylet, three-way stopcock, manometer (long, hollow calibrated rod), and collecting devices for CSF specimens.

PREPARATION   None.

TECHNIQUE   A. Position
The patient lies in a lateral recumbent position with his back at the edge of the examining table, knees drawn up to the abdomen and head flexed onto the chest (Fig. 2-1). This position widens the space between the spinous processes of the lower lumbar vertebrae so that the needle

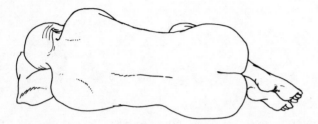

Figure 2-1. Position for lumbar puncture. Head is flexed onto chest and knees are drawn up to the abdomen.

can easily enter between them. The assistant must help the patient to assume and maintain this position. Physical and emotional relaxation of the patient while in position is of paramount importance, as anxiety and resultant muscle tension may cause falsely elevated pressure readings, and tensing of back muscles makes positioning of the needle difficult. Relaxation can be facilitated by having the patient breathe slowly and deeply through the mouth.

Occasionally, when puncture is difficult to perform with the patient lying on his side, he will be seated on the bed, leaning forward on a table. Once successful puncture is accomplished the procedure is completed either with the patient seated or after he has been assisted to lie down on his side.

B. Procedure

The appropriate intervertebral space is located by palpation of bony landmarks. The area is cleansed with an antiseptic solution, the surrounding area draped with sterile towels, and the needle puncture site usually infiltrated with a local anesthetic. The needle is inserted between the spinous processes and laminae into the spinal canal and subarachnoid space (Fig. 2-2). The stylet is removed and a good flow of CSF is established. A manometer is attached to the needle for pressure recordings. Once the needle is in place, the assistant may be asked to help the patient straighten his legs and extend his head slightly to a more comfortable position. CSF is allowed to enter the manometer by manipulating the stopcock

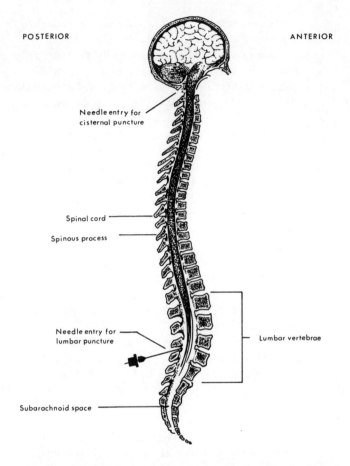

POSTERIOR

ANTERIOR

Needle entry for
cisternal puncture

Spinal cord

Spinous process

Needle entry for
lumbar puncture

Lumbar vertebrae

Subarachnoid space

Figure 2-2. Lateral view of the spinal column and vertebrae showing the level at which the spinal cord ends and the needle entry sites for lumbar and cisternal punctures.

handle, and the pressure is measured at the point where the fluid stops rising and fluctuates within a limited range. This is the opening pressure (normal is 60 to 180 mm of water in the lateral recumbent position). Between 5 and 10 ml of CSF is usually removed for laboratory investigation. A final pressure reading is obtained, and the needle is withdrawn. A Band-Aid may be applied to the puncture site.

If the patient is attached to a respirator, the value of CSF pressure becomes artificially elevated. Therefore the respirator may need to be temporarily disconnected during the measurement to obtain a more accurate value.

When spinal cord compression is suspected, the Queckenstedt test may be performed during the lumbar puncture. After the opening pressure is ascertained, compression is applied to the veins of the neck either manually or by means of a blood pressure cuff wrapped around the patient's neck and inflated to 40 mm of mercury. There are several variations of this maneuver. The normal end result should be a rapid rise in the pressure level in the manometer and then a return to the previous reading within seconds after the cuff is deflated. If the pressure does not fall back, this is usually indicative of a block to free flow of CSF in the spinal subarachnoid space.

PATIENT SENSATIONS

When the local anesthetic is injected, the patient will feel the sting of the needle as in a venipuncture, followed shortly by a feeling of numbness at the injection site. There is a sensation of pressure rather than pain as the lumbar puncture needle is inserted. If there is difficulty in placing the needle, a spinal nerve may be inadvertently stimulated, causing sharp pain to radiate down one leg or into the buttock or groin. When this occurs the physician immediately pulls back on the needle and redirects its course. It is of utmost importance to reassure the patient that no harm has been done and that the needle is being inserted well below the end of the spinal cord itself and will cause no damage.

AFTERCARE

1. The physician usually requires that the patient remain flat in bed for 4 to 24 hours. Any position is acceptable as long as the head is not higher than the rest of the body.
2. Extra fluid intake should be encouraged to help replace the fluid removed.
3. Some patients may develop a headache following a lumbar puncture. This is more frequent when it has been necessary to make several attempts to enter the subarachnoid space and a rent in the dura and arachnoid allows continued

loss of CSF after the needle has been removed. The site of the leak cannot be seen, as it lies deep in the tissues of the back and the CSF is absorbed into the surrounding tissues. It does not exit through the puncture site. The headache usually begins within 30 minutes after the patient first sits up and is often characterized by pain in the occiput and neck. Lying flat and the use of analgesics will help to relieve it. The headache usually persists for only 24 hours but occasionally may linger for a week or more.

4. The patient should be observed for any deterioration in neurological status.

Cisternal Puncture

PURPOSE
Withdrawal of cerebrospinal fluid (CSF) by insertion of a thin hollow needle between the foramen magnum and the first cervical vertebra into the subarachnoid space (see Fig. 2-2).
This procedure is usually performed:
1. When lumbar puncture is not possible owing to bony abnormalities or an abnormally low spinal cord.
2. With a lumbar puncture to demonstrate the upper limits of a block in the spinal subarachnoid space.

TIME
Ten to 30 minutes.

LOCATION
Patient's room or treatment room.

PERSONNEL
Physician and assistant.

EQUIPMENT
A hollow needle (shorter than that used for a lumbar puncture) with stylet, three-way stopcock, manometer (long, hollow calibrated rod), collecting devices for CSF specimens, and shaving equipment.

PREPARATION
The nape of the patient's neck is shaved in the midline up to the occipital protuberance.

TECHNIQUE
1. The patient is placed in a lateral position on the edge of the bed or treatment table; the head is supported on a pillow with the chin flexed onto the chest. This position makes the puncture site more accessible by bringing the brain stem and cord forward in the spinal canal, providing more room posteriorly for needle entry.
2. After the skin is cleansed with an antiseptic solution and locally anesthetized, the surrounding area is draped with sterile towels and the needle inserted.

3. Opening and closing pressures are measured, and CSF is removed for laboratory analysis as with a lumbar puncture (see page 17).

PATIENT
SENSATIONS

The patient will experience:
1. Discomfort from maintaining the required position, especially if he is elderly or arthritic.
2. A stinging sensation during injection of the local anesthetic.
3. Dull pressure at the puncture site as the needle is inserted.

AFTERCARE

1. The needle enters the cisterna magna, which overlies the cerebellum and lower medulla where cardiorespiratory centers are located. Therefore the patient must be observed for signs of sudden respiratory distress and changes in blood pressure and pulse both *during* and after the procedure.
2. The patient should be observed for any deterioration in neurological status.
3. If the procedure is done on an outpatient basis, the patient may return home only after it has been clearly established by observation of neurological status and vital signs that there are no untoward sequelae.
4. Continued CSF leakage, with subsequent development of headache, is rare, making bed rest unnecessary.
5. The patient should be encouraged to increase fluid intake to facilitate CSF replacement.

Pneumoencephalography (PEG)

PURPOSE   Visualization of the cerebral ventricular system (Fig. 2-3) and subarachnoid space to:
1. Localize or define a mass lesion, or both.
2. Demonstrate loss of brain substance.
3. Demonstrate obstruction of normal cerebrospinal fluid (CSF) pathways.

TIME   Two to 4 hours.

LOCATION   Radiology department.

PERSONNEL   Physician and assistants.

EQUIPMENT   Lumbar or cisternal puncture tray (see pages 15, 20), somersaulting chair (Fig. 2-4), and fluoroscopy unit.*

TECHNIQUE   1. An intravenous infusion may be started before the procedure is begun to maintain hydration and help prevent hypotension. It also provides an immediate route should intravenous medication be necessary.
2. The patient is securely positioned in the somersaulting chair so that he is entirely immobilized. Prevention of head movement is important for obtaining good visualization as well as decreasing headache and nausea during the procedure.
3. A lumbar or cisternal puncture is performed after the puncture site has been cleansed with an antiseptic solution,

---

*A fluoroscope with image intensification, spot film device, and television monitor. A fluoroscope is a device which employs x-rays without recording the image on film. It is used most often to visualize physiological motion, such as swallowing function. Image intensification increases the clarity of the fluoroscopic image on the television monitor by enhancing its brightness. Spot films are made as the patient is being fluoroscoped and provide a permanent record of significant events.

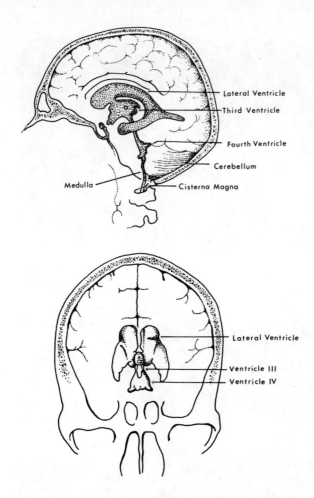

Figure 2-3. Cerebral ventricular system (*top*, lateral view; *bottom*, anterior view).

the area draped with sterile towels, and the skin infiltrated with a local anesthetic.

4. A small amount of CSF is withdrawn and may be sent for laboratory determinations. Small increments of sterile gas are slowly injected through the needle. Since the gas is lighter than CSF it rises into the ventricular system. The different densities of the gas and CSF provide the contrast needed for the x-ray films.

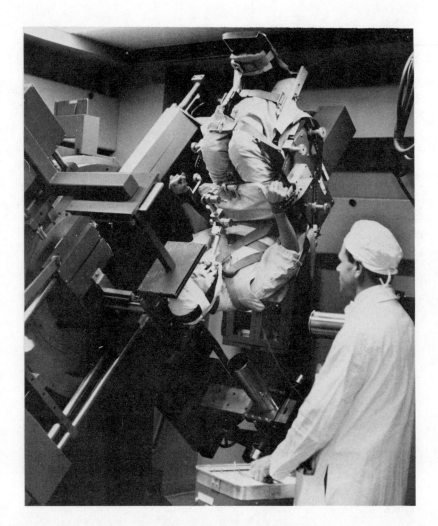

Figure 2-4. Somersaulting chair used for pneumoencephalography. (Courtesy Columbia-Presbyterian Medical Center, New York.)

5. After gas placement is verified fluoroscopically, appropriate films are taken with the patient upright in the chair.
6. Once all the necessary views in this position have been taken, the chair is rotated forward slowly until a 360-

degree turn has been made. Rotation of the chair and gravity cause the gas to be shifted from one area to another, thereby gradually opacifying the entire cerebral ventricular system and the subarachnoid space. Spot films are taken depending on what is seen fluoroscopically.

7. When all the necessary films have been taken the patient is returned to an upright position, the needle removed, and the puncture site covered with a Band-Aid.

8. Throughout the procedure and at its completion the patient's neurological and cardiovascular status is evaluated.

PREPARATION
1. All foods and fluids are usually withheld before the procedure for the following reasons:
   a. To minimize the danger of emesis and aspiration in a procedure which usually causes nausea and requires immobilization of the patient's head throughout.
   b. Because craniotomy may be necessary immediately after the procedure.

2. The back of the head may be shaved if a cisternal puncture is planned.

3. Neurological and cardiovascular status is evaluated. The values are recorded to establish a baseline for post-procedural evaluation.

4. Elastic stockings or Ace bandages may be applied to both legs to prevent the hypotension that is sometimes a complication of the dependent position of the legs and the rotation of the chair.

5. Dentures should be removed.

6. Hair should be clean, unbraided, unmatted, and free of hair preparations to prevent extraneous shadows from appearing on the films.

7. All hairpins, necklaces, and other metal objects which might appear on the films and obscure significant anatomical structures should be removed.

8. Premedication is administered to produce maximum relaxation and cooperation in the patient without impairing his ability to respond to directions and evaluative questions during the procedure.

**PATIENT
SENSATIONS**

1. Fear of the somersaulting chair should be anticipated. Assure the patient that he will be securely supported and there is no danger of falling despite rotation.
2. Fear of the lumbar or cisternal puncture part of the procedure should be dealt with as suggested in those procedures (see pages 18, 19, 21).
3. The patient will experience a stinging sensation when the local anesthetic is administered and dull pressure when the lumbar or cisternal puncture needle is inserted.
4. The patient will experience what may be the most excruciating headache of his life, associated with severe nausea. In spite of this great pain, no damage is being done, and once he lies down at the end of the procedure, the headache will be substantially less. During the procedure he will have to follow the instructions of the physician as to placement of his head; a sudden movement of the head can move the air into the wrong places, and more air will have to be added.
5. The patient therefore should report any headache, nausea, faintness, respiratory distress, or other untoward sensation experienced during the procedure.

AFTERCARE

For the first 24 hours after the procedure the patient must be evaluated frequently in relation to the preprocedure baseline. Particular attention must be paid to any alterations in mentation, alertness, and pupillary size and reactivity. Additional neurological signs indicative of motor and sensory status as well as vital signs should also be assessed.

Headache, nausea, vomiting, and elevated temperature are the most common sequelae of pneumoencephalography and should receive appropriate intervention. Fluid intake should be encouraged and the patient maintained flat in bed for the first 24 to 48 hours to minimize the possibility or severity of complications. Most of these symptoms should subside within this 24- to 48-hour period.

Myelography

PURPOSE   Visualization of the spinal subarachnoid space to define it and to evaluate lesions involving neural elements.

TIME   Approximately 2 hours.

LOCATION   Radiology department.

PERSONNEL   Radiologist and assistants.

EQUIPMENT   Lumbar or cisternal puncture tray (see pages 15, 20), fluoroscopy unit, and x-ray table. The special myelography x-ray table (Fig. 2-5) has straps and shoulder and foot supports to secure the patient's position on the table. This ensures comfort and prevents slipping when the table is tilted. Most tables have hand grips which the patient may grasp.

TECHNIQUE   1. The initial step in myelography is the performance of a lumbar or cisternal puncture either above or below the site of a suspected lesion. In addition to the usual lateral position, the puncture may be done with the patient sitting or lying prone. Appropriate placement of the needle is verified fluoroscopically and by the appearance of cerebrospinal fluid (CSF) dripping from the needle. A small amount of CSF is removed to allow its replacement by the contrast material.* Specimens may be sent for laboratory determinations.
2. After placing the patient in a prone position, the radiologist injects the contrast material into the sub-

---

*The injection or ingestion of a contrast agent creates an alteration in tissue density. This is achieved by the use of either a gas, which is a negative contrast agent, or a positive contrast agent such as barium. Negative agents permit the passage of radiation through them, while positive mediums absorb radiation. Both provide a contrast with surrounding tissues.

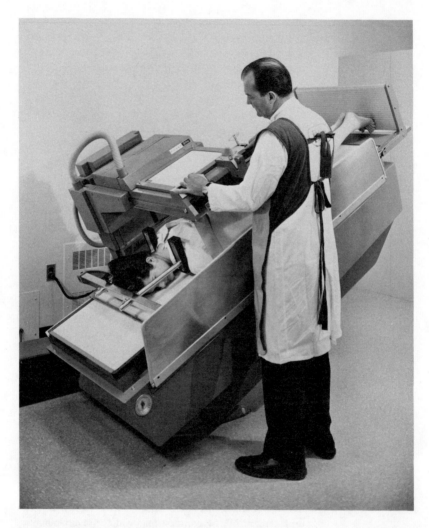

Figure 2-5. Special myelography table, with straps and supports to prevent the patient from slipping when the table is tilted. (Courtesy Picker Corporation, Cleveland, Ohio.)

arachnoid space. An oily contrast medium is usually employed. It is heavier than CSF and does not mix with it; therefore it can be manipulated by gravity into any area of the spinal subarachnoid space. For examination of the cervical or thoracic spine the head of the x-ray table is tilted down; conversely, for examination of the lower lumbar region, the foot of the table is tilted down.

3. Appropriate radiographs are taken depending on what is seen fluoroscopically. These may be multiple in number and include different projections. In order to obtain most of these films, the x-ray apparatus is maneuvered. Sometimes the patient, too, must be repositioned, but usually only to a slightly oblique angle.

4. When the study has been completed, the x-ray table is tilted to cause the contrast material to collect around the puncture needle. The contrast material is removed by allowing it to drip out through the needle or by withdrawing it with a syringe. The table is then leveled, the needle withdrawn, and a Band-Aid placed over the puncture site.

PREPARATION
1. The patient is usually kept NPO before the procedure as nausea and vomiting may result from either the lumbar or cisternal puncture or the tilting of the table.

2. A baseline record of vital signs and neurological status (especially motor and sensory) should be obtained before the patient is premedicated to provide a means for postprocedure comparison.

3. All metal items, such as jewelry and safety pins, should be removed from the area to be studied to prevent extraneous shadows from appearing on the films.

4. A sedative is administered beforehand to control anxiety and thus enable the patient more easily to tolerate a lengthy, tiring, and uncomfortable procedure. Atropine is often given to counteract the vagal effect resulting from changes in position during myelography.

PATIENT SENSATIONS
The patient may experience:

1. The discomfort of a lumbar puncture (see page 18) or cisternal puncture (see page 21) and the accompanying injection of a local anesthetic.

2. Fear of slipping on the tilting table. This should be allayed by explanation of the efforts made to position

the patient safely and comfortably. The patient should report any sensation of slipping.

3. Sweating, dizziness, faintness, nausea, and vomiting from the changes in positions on the tilt table. This is sometimes related to the speed at which the table is tilted. Therefore the patient should report any untoward sensations so that corrective measures may be initiated.

4. Sharp, stabbing, radiating pain during removal of the contrast material if suction with a syringe is applied.

5. Sensations of headache, nausea, and back pain during the first 24 hours, although they may persist for as long as a week.

AFTERCARE

1. Neurological status and vital signs should be determined immediately upon the patient's return to the unit and at frequent intervals thereafter. Particular attention should be paid to motor and sensory status and note made of any alterations from the baseline. As urinary retention is sometimes a postprocedure problem, secondary to an alteration in dynamics or irritation by the contrast medium, special note should be made of the time and amount of the patient's voiding.

2. To obviate the development of headache or nausea, or both, the patient is kept flat in bed for 24 hours.

3. Fluid intake should be encouraged to assist in replacement of the CSF and rehydration.

4. Infrequently the patient may develop a stiff neck and mild fever secondary to chemical meningitis. The modesty of the signs and temperature elevation and the clinical appearance help to distinguish this from infectious meningitis, although only smears and cultures can definitely rule out the latter.

5. Sometimes the dye is not completely removed, either because it becomes technically too difficult to remove it, or because it continues to settle into pockets not visualized on the first day. Such patients, when returned to their bed, must not at any time let their back be higher than their head, since the dye may then run into the head and be irretrievable. Dye removal may then be attempted in the myelography room the day after the original procedure.

Angiography of the Head and Neck

PURPOSE   Visualization of the cerebral vasculature or its extracranial
sources, or both, to:
    a. Evaluate abnormalities of vascular structure and function.
    b. Identify mass lesions by observation of vessel displace-
ment and areas of abnormal vascularity.

TIME   Thirty minutes to 3 hours. Variables determining time
include the age of the patient, the status of the vasculature,
and the problem under investigation.

LOCATION   Radiology department.

PERSONNEL   Radiologist and assistants.

EQUIPMENT   Standard x-ray table, rapid-sequence film changer or cineradiograph, and fluoroscopy unit.

PREPARATION 1. When a femoral or axillary puncture is to be performed,
the groin or axilla is shaved and scrubbed with an antiseptic
solution. Some institutions prefer to have both groins or
axillae thus prepared in case of difficulty of access on one
side.
2. The patient is kept fasting. Hydration is usually maintained, either orally or intravenously, before the procedure to prevent excessive concentration of the contrast
material in the cerebral vasculature, which could cause
neurological deterioration.
3. Dentures should be removed.
4. All hairpins, necklaces, and other metal objects which
might appear on the films and obscure significant
anatomical structures should be removed.
5. Hair should be clean, unbraided, unmatted, and free of
any preparation to prevent extraneous shadows from
appearing on the films.

31

6. As this procedure may be lengthy the patient should void before leaving the unit. Accommodating the patient's desire to void during the procedure may be logistically difficult.
7. A baseline record of vital signs and neurological status should be obtained before the patient is premedicated to provide a means of comparison after the procedure.
8. A sedative, tranquilizer, or analgesic, or any combination thereof, is administered to relax the patient effectively without hindering his ability to cooperate and respond to evaluative questions during the procedure. Further premedication may include atropine to reduce possible effects of irritation of the carotid sinus.

TECHNIQUE

Opacification of the extracranial or cerebral vasculature or both can be achieved by various means, depending on the clinical problem, the preference and experience of the investigator, and the available facilities. Direct needle puncture of the artery, usually the common carotid or brachial, is frequently used.

Selective percutaneous needle puncture of a distant artery, such as the femoral, followed by the introduction of a flexible radiopaque catheter which is advanced to the vessel under investigation is another common method. The aortic arch and its main branches supplying the brain may be studied in this manner.

1. The procedure begins by placing the patient in a supine position on the x-ray table. If for any reason the patient is unable to cooperate, restraints may be applied to prevent inadvertent contamination or dislodgment of the needle or catheter. An intravenous infusion may be started at this time if it has not already been, to maintain hydration and to provide an easily accessible route for medication.
2. The skin over the puncture site is cleansed with an antiseptic solution and infiltrated with a local anesthetic, and the adjacent areas are covered with sterile drapes.
3. For the direct puncture technique, the desired vessel is located by palpation and the needle is directly inserted.

If the carotid artery is the vessel to be punctured, it is imperative that the patient's head be absolutely motionless. A restraint may be used to achieve this immobilization. For selective percutaneous needle puncture, the artery is punctured, and the catheter is advanced under fluoroscopic guidance into the vessel or vessels to be studied.

4. Usually a small amount of the contrast material is injected and a preliminary film obtained to ensure proper placement of the needle or catheter.

5. When the needle is appropriately placed, the contrast material is rapidly injected and recorded either cineradiographically or by exposing multiple films in rapid sequence. The films taken will demonstrate all phases of circulation — aterial, capillary, and venous. If special views are desired, minor changes in the position of the patient's head may be required.

6. If the radiologist wishes to study more than one vessel by the selective catheterization method, further injections will be necessary. An interval of 10 to 15 minutes is required before this can be done. During this time the catheter is repositioned under fluoroscopic guidance. Several such repositionings may be necessary if an extensive study is necessary. As each vessel is opacified, further filming is done.

   If the direct puncture technique is used and more than one vessel is to be studied, each one is punctured separately.

7. When the areas supplied by the carotid artery are being studied, the radiologist may elect to perform a cross-compression test. The test is performed by having an assistant apply pressure to the carotid artery on the side opposite that being studied. This should demonstrate whether the carotid artery on the uncompressed side is capable of supplying adequate circulation to the opposite cerebral hemisphere. This test may obviate the necessity for bilateral examinations.

8. Throughout the procedure the patient is observed for any neurological deterioration. Cardiovascular status is also evaluated by obtaining frequent blood pressure

readings and by electrocardiographic monitoring. Any major alterations may require immediate cessation of the procedure and institution of appropriate corrective measures.

9. At the completion of the angiographic study, the needle or catheter is withdrawn and firm pressure applied to the puncture site for approximately 15 minutes. The area is observed carefully to ensure that there is no bleeding from the puncture site and that distal pulses are full before the patient is returned to his room. The patient's cardiovascular and neurological condition is evaluated again, as it has been throughout the procedure.

PATIENT SENSATIONS

The patient may experience:

1. A burning sensation from injection of the local anesthetic.
2. Discomfort from maintaining one position for an extended period of time on a hard surface.
3. Discomfort and frustration if restraints have been applied.
4. Pain from the contrast material, the intensity varying with the artery injected. Carotid injections often cause a transient burning or painful sensation in the head or behind the eyes; brachial injections produce a severe burning sensation in the arm, shoulder, and base of the neck.
5. Transient nausea and headache during injection of the contrast material.
6. Embarrassment from the preprocedure shaving of the groin and from the brief exposure of the groin area prior to placement of the drapes.
7. Postprocedure discomfort at the puncture site; or pain if a hematoma develops.

AFTERCARE

1. Irritation of the cerebral vessels by the contrast material or from manipulation of the needle or catheter during the procedure may lead to deterioration in the patient's neurological status. This may also occur as the result of hematoma or embolization to a distal cerebral artery if the puncture site was in the carotid or vertebral vessels. The patient should be observed for:

a. Changes in level of consciousness, such as restlessness, confusion, disorientation, or lethargy.

b. Motor or sensory deterioration, such as extremity weakness, decreased position sense or response to pain, or inequality in pupillary size and reactivity to light.

c. Appearance of seizure activity.

d. Elevation in blood pressure with a concomitant widening pulse pressure, a slow pulse, and altered respirations, all signs of increased intracranial pressure.

2. Arrhythmias may occur if there has been excessive irritation of the carotid sinus during carotid angiography.

3. Blood pressure determinations should not be obtained in the arm in which an axillary or brachial puncture was done.

4. A cold pack should be applied to decrease the possibility of hematoma formation.

5. Particular attention must be paid to a puncture site in the neck. A hematoma in the neck may cause compression on the trachea and larynx and if not noted early may lead to respiratory embarrassment.

6. If bleeding or swelling is evident at the puncture site, manual pressure should be applied and medical assistance summoned immediately.

7. Signs of decreased or occluded peripheral circulation will develop if there is embolization to a distal artery from, or hematoma formation at, a puncture site in an extremity. Therefore the presence of peripheral pulses should be ascertained frequently and compared with the baseline. In addition, the color and temperature of the involved extremity should be noted.

8. The patient remains in bed for the period specified, usually 12 to 24 hours. If the puncture was made in the groin or antecubital fossa, the hip or elbow is immobilized in extension.

Electroencephalography (EEG)

PURPOSE   Detection and localization of abnormal electrical activity in the brain.

TIME   Forty-five to 60 minutes for a routine EEG. Three hours or more for a sleep EEG.

LOCATION   Electroencephalography suite. A portable EEG machine is available for critically ill patients.

PERSONNEL   Technician.

EQUIPMENT   Stretcher or chair, EEG console (Fig. 2-6), and electrodes (Fig. 2-7).

TECHNIQUE   With the patient lying down or seated in a chair, the technician either secures standard electrodes to the patient's scalp with collodion or paste or inserts needle electrodes subcutaneously. This is to ensure airtight contact and therefore minimize interference with the recording. The electrodes are evenly distributed over the entire scalp. Placement requires approximately 15 minutes.

The patient is instructed to lie quietly with his eyes closed. Any movement, including that of the eyes, will interfere with the accuracy of the recording. As each electrode is attached to a separate pen on the electroencephalograph, the recording demonstrates the electrical activity of the brain surface beneath each electrode.

Modifications of this technique may be done to supplement information gained from the routine EEG.

1. Nasopharyngeal electrodes (long, curved metal probes) are placed in the nostrils to obtain otherwise inaccessible inferior and medial temporal lobe recordings. This may be quite uncomfortable, particularly for the patient with a deviated septum or swollen turbinates.

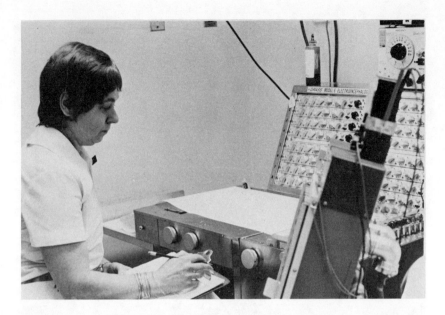

Figure 2-6. Electroencephalographic console. (Courtesy Lucy B. Lazzopina, Columbia-Presbyterian Medical Center, New York.)

2. Activation techniques are methods by which abnormal electrical activity may be elicited more easily and recorded.
   a. The patient is asked to hyperventilate.
   b. Flashing (strobe) lights are directed into the patient's eyes at varying rates.
   c. The patient is medicated with a hypnotic to induce sleep. The sleep EEG is used to elicit temporal lobe foci or to lateralize or localize abnormalities which were diffuse while the patient was awake. It may also be used to evoke abnormal sleep patterns. This technique will necessarily extend the length of the procedure since recording cannot begin until the patient is asleep.
   d. Pentylenetetrazol (Metrazol), a stimulant, is administered intravenously to induce subclinical seizure activity, thereby localizing a lesion.

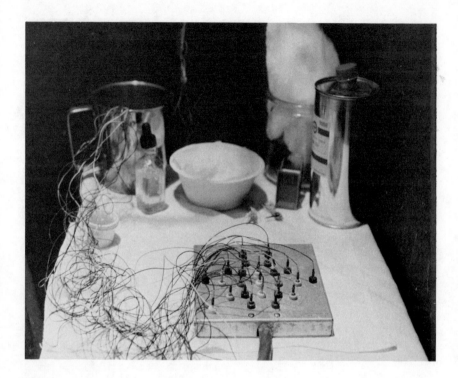

Figure 2-7. Electroencephalographic electrodes and equipment for securing and removing them.

PREPARATION

1. Anticonvulsants usually are not discontinued for this study.
2. The patient should have clean hair, free of any preparations. If collodion or paste is used to attach the electrodes, clean hair provides good contact; if needle electrodes are used, the possibility of infection is minimized.
3. Hairpins, barrettes, clips, ribbons, wigs, and toupees must be removed.
4. The patient should be reassured that no electrical shock will be experienced during this procedure.
5. As hypoglycemia in itself may produce an abnormal EEG, the patient should be instructed to eat before the procedure.

PATIENT
SENSATIONS

1. During hyperventilation, the patient may feel dizzy or light-headed.
2. If needle electrodes are employed, the patient may experience a feeling like that of a single hair's being pulled with a placement of each electrode. Patients with a thick layer of fat beneath the skin usually feel nothing. Persons who have undergone the test have noted "hearing" the electrode go through the skin. Neither sensation is experienced as painful.

AFTERCARE

1. After the collodion has dried, removal may be facilitated by brushing the hair vigorously. The remainder of the collodion can be removed with careful use of a solvent such as acetone. Hair washing will complete the cleansing process.
2. If a sleep EEG has been performed on an outpatient, someone should accompany the patient home, as the hypnotic will not have worn off completely. If the patient is hospitalized, he can be expected to sleep for several hours after returning to the unit.

Electromyography (EMG) and Nerve and Muscle Stimulation

PURPOSE
: Evaluation of muscle and nerve electrical activity to determine the presence of neuromuscular abnormalities, including disorders of the spinal cord, peripheral nerves, and muscles.

TIME
: One to 2 1/2 hours.

LOCATION
: Diagnostic suite.

PERSONNEL
: Technician or physician for nerve and muscle stimulation; physician for needle electromyography.

EQUIPMENT
: Electrodes, oscilloscope, amplifier and loudspeaker, camera, and electrical stimulator.

PREPARATION
: 1. For patients who are unable to cooperate or have a low pain threshold, adequate sedation or analgesia, or both, are essential.
2. Muscle serum enzyme levels must be determined prior to electromyography since the latter will cause misleading elevation of these chemical values for up to 10 days.
3. This study is usually done prior to myelography and muscle biopsy, as these procedures may be better planned once the results of the electromyographic study are known.

TECHNIQUE
: For this procedure the patient is placed in a supine position. There are two parts to the examination.
A. Nerve conduction
Peripheral nerves are stimulated at superficial points, usually in the limbs, and the resulting muscle and nerve electrical activity is recorded. Normally, surface electrodes are used and repetitive stimulation rates of up to 20 impulses per second may be required.

B. Needle electromyography

A single small needle (an insulated wire 1/2 to 3 inches long) is inserted into the muscle to be studied. The number and location of muscles sampled depend on the clinical problem, but as many as ten or more insertions may be made. The needle is advanced into the muscle by increments. At each level observations are made of the electrical activity during the following conditions:

1. On insertion.
2. At rest.
3. During gentle voluntary muscle contraction.
4. During maximal voluntary effort.

The electrical activity consists of motor unit potentials of about 0.001 volt which are magnified by the amplifier and viewed on the oscilloscope screen. Sound equivalents are heard on the loudspeaker. Permanent recordings are obtained on film or on a fiberoptic paper graph and can be stored on magnetic tape.

PATIENT SENSATIONS

1. A brief, sharp pain will be experienced as each needle is inserted and advanced into the muscle. This is usually much less than the pain associated with an intramuscular injection.
2. The electrical stimulation will cause an intermittent tingling sensation similar to the shocks one receives from static electricity. It is not usually regarded as significantly painful if appropriately explained and only small, innocuous currents are used.
3. During the procedure the electrical activity from the muscle can be heard over the loudspeaker as a crackling, harsh sound similar to that of thunder. The volume of the sound can be modulated by the examiner.

AFTERCARE

The points of needle insertion are compressed for at least 30 seconds to avoid the rare possibility of hematoma formation.

Computerized Transaxial Tomography (CTT) (CAT Scan)

PURPOSE
To visualize, define, and precisely localize intracranial lesions.

This is a new diagnostic radiological procedure that is quickly gaining support. Its advantages are early detection of intracranial abnormalities and ease in following the course and management of intracranial disease. It is a safe, noninvasive procedure and easily tolerated by the patient.

TIME
Thirty minutes.

LOCATION
Radiology department.

PERSONNEL
Radiologist and technician.

EQUIPMENT
Examination table, EMI scanner, viewing screen, computer, printout device, and Polaroid camera.

PREPARATION
Immobility is essential to ensure accurate pictures. If the patient cannot fully cooperate, sedation may be given.

TECHNIQUE
The x-ray tube beam makes a 180-degree scan of the head, 1 degree at a time, in three or four different planes. It records the absorption coefficients of different tissues at different planes through the head. The tissue densities are arbitrarily assigned numbers (absorption coefficients) ranging from −500 for air to +500 for bone. When the scan is completed, the computer supplies a printout of the absorption coefficients presented in a fashion that corresponds to the shape of the plane of the head studied (Fig. 2-8a).

Photographs are taken of the image on the screen (Fig. 2-8b). Air appears on the picture as black, bone as white. Soft tissues are in the 0 to +20 range and therefore appear as shades of gray.

The pattern of shades and their correlation to different tissue densities in the brain assist in identifying the nature of an abnormality. Furthermore, because each scan is of a specific plane, the additional dimension of depth is added. This allows more precise localization of the abnormality within the cranium.

1. The patient lies in a supine position on a padded examination table with his head extending into the scanning unit (Fig. 2-9). Surrounding the head (from the forehead to the occiput) is a rubber diaphragm which separates the patient from a box containing water. The diaphragm is adjusted to fit snugly. This provides an air-free path for the x-ray beam, ensuring a more accurate reading.
2. If a lesion is noticed but cannot be clearly identified, small amounts of a contrast medium are injected intravenously. This material intensifies the absorption densities of the abnormality, particularly if it is highly vascular. The increased tissue density produces better delineation of the abnormal area.
3. The supine position is maintained throughout the study.

PATIENT SENSATIONS   None.

AFTERCARE   None.

A

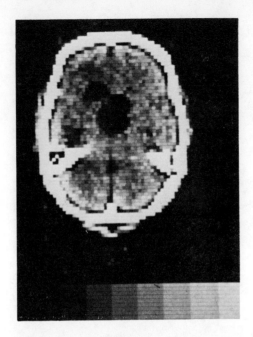

B

Figure 2-8. Cystic craniopharyngioma demonstrated by means of computerized transaxial tomography. **A.** Computer printout of absorption coefficients. **B.** Polaroid photograph of EMI scan. (Courtesy EMI Electronics and Industrial Operations, Hayes, England.)

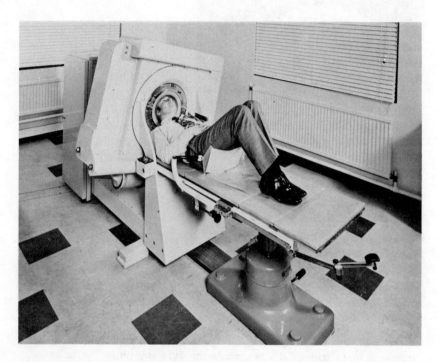

Figure 2-9. Patient positioned for EMI scan. (Courtesy EMI Electronics and Industrial Operations, Hayes, England.)

Bibliography

Ambrose, J. Computerized x-ray scanning of the brain. *J. Neurosurg.* 40:679, 1974.

Baker, A. B. (Ed.). *Clinical Neurology* (3d ed.). Hagerstown, Md.: Harper & Row, 1973.

Baker, H. L., et al. Computer assisted tomography of the head and early evaluation. *Mayo Clin. Proc.* 49:17, 1974.

Bickerstaff, E. R. *Neurology for Nurses* (2d ed.). London: English Universities Press, 1971.

Carini, E., and Owens, G. *Neurological and Neurosurgical Nursing* (5th ed.). St. Louis: Mosby, 1970.

Chusid, J. G. *Correlative Neuroanatomy and Functional Neurology* (15th ed.). Los Altos, Calif.: Lange, 1973.

Fields, W. S., et al. Special procedures and equipment in the diagnosis and management of stroke. *Stroke* 4:113, 1973.

New, P. F. J., et al. Computerized axial tomography with the EMI scanner. *Radiology* 110:1091, 1974.

Taveras, J. M., et al. *Diagnostic Neuroradiology* (2d ed.). Baltimore: Williams & Wilkins, 1973.

Toole, J. F. (Ed.). *Special Techniques for Neurological Diagnosis.* Philadelphia: Davis, 1969.

Youmans, J. R. (Ed.). *Neurological Surgery,* Vol. 1. Philadelphia: Saunders, 1973.

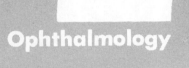

Ophthalmology

3

Visual Acuity

PURPOSE   Evaluation of visual acuity.

TIME   Fifteen minutes. If the patient has poor vision or difficulty in cooperating, the procedure will necessarily be longer.

LOCATION   Any area that is well illuminated and permits the patient to sit or stand 20 feet away from the chart.

PERSONNEL   Physician, nurse, or trained assistant.

EQUIPMENT   The Snellen chart, which consists of letters and numbers in gradually decreasing sizes. Each row of letters is assigned a number corresponding to the distance in feet from the chart at which that particular sized letter can be seen by the normal eye. Therefore someone with 20/40 vision is able to see at 20 feet those letters on the row assigned the number 40. The higher the number assigned, the larger the letters are.

PREPARATION   If the patient wears glasses, he should be instructed to bring them with him as they are a necessary part of the examination.

TECHNIQUE
1. The patient faces the chart at a distance of 20 feet.
2. Eyeglasses are removed.
3. With one eye covered, the patient is asked to identify the letters or numbers on the chart as pointed out by the examiner.
4. With the opposite eye covered, the procedure is repeated.
5. The procedure will be repeated with the patient wearing his glasses to evaluate the degree to which they correct his vision.

PATIENT
SENSATIONS   None.

AFTERCARE   Corrective lenses as necessary.

Perimetry
(Visual Field Examination)

PURPOSE   Evaluation of the peripheral field of vision to determine the function of the retina, optic nerve, and optic pathways to detect lesions of the eye and brain.

TIME   Usually 20 to 30 minutes. If the patient has difficulty in cooperating, the time period may be considerably lengthened in the effort to obtain accurate results.

LOCATION   Examining room. A preliminary evaluation without special equipment can be done at the bedside.

PERSONNEL   Physician or technician.

ROOM AND EQUIPMENT   Dimly lit room, large black screen with central dot (tangent screen), 2 spotlights, test objects such as a small light or round target object on a pointer, and table with mounted support against which the patient rests his head.

PREPARATION   If the patient wears glasses, he should be instructed to bring them to the examination.

TECHNIQUE   The patient is seated in the chair at a predetermined distance from the tangent screen (approximately 3 feet). His head rests on and is stabilized by supports at the chin and forehead. Since head immobility is important, a light metal brace extending from the forehead back to the upper occiput is sometimes applied to ensure complete stability.

With glasses on, if usually worn, the patient is directed to fix his eyes on the object at the center of the screen and to gaze at it steadily without deviation throughout the examination. This requires concentration and ability to cooperate, and is essential to accurate testing. The spotlights, which are positioned on either side of the patient and directed at the screen to ensure its visibility in the dimly lit room, are turned off at some time during the examination. Each eye is tested separately. While one is being examined, the other is covered.

A small dot of light or a small target object on a black pointer is moved by degrees and from various angles into the patient's field of vision from the periphery. The patient is instructed to tell the examiner when the object is first seen or when it moves. Each of these points is marked on the screen by a black pin, gradually establishing a pattern which is later transferred to a graph chart of the eye fields.

Frequently the technician will repeat maneuvers to verify the patient's initial response.

PATIENT SENSATIONS

Fear of what the examination may reveal often puts severe stress on the patient, which may cause him to be less than honest in his responses. It is important to emphasize that he respond as accurately and honestly as possible. This is crucial for the patient's welfare, as it is necessary for making an accurate diagnosis and choosing appropriate therapy.

AFTERCARE

None.

Pupil Dilatation

PURPOSE   Production of mydriasis (dilation of the pupil) and cycloplegia (paralysis of accommodation) to facilitate examination of the eye.

TIME   Thirty to 45 minutes.

LOCATION   Patient's room, treatment room, or physician's office.

PERSONNEL   Nurse, technician, or physician.

EQUIPMENT   Mydriatic-cycloplegic eye drops such as cyclopentolate hydrochloride (Cyclogyl), eyedropper, and tissues.

TECHNIQUE   One drop of the solution is instilled 2 times with a 5-minute interval. For rapid dilation, the drops may be instilled at a shorter interval.

PREPARATION   The outpatient should arrange to have someone accompany him home following the procedure since vision will be transiently impaired. Driving will not be possible during this time.

PATIENT SENSATIONS AND AFTERCARE
1. The eye drops may sting or burn as they are instilled. The patient may also have what is described as a "funny taste" in his mouth. Both sensations are transitory and will cease when the dilatation procedure is completed.
2. Because of the effects of the eye drops, patients will be unable to react normally to changes in light intensity or to focus on nearby objects. Therefore vision will be impaired, precluding reading, driving, and similar activities until the effects have worn off. Bright lights will be very irritating. Dark glasses will alleviate this discomfort to some extent. The local effects of these drugs persist for several hours after their application.

3. Particularly in elderly people, the administration of mydriatics can precipitate acute glaucoma, an ophthalmological emergency.
4. Rarely mydriatic agents may produce transitory untoward systemic effects, including dryness of the mouth, flushing, dizziness, and tachycardia.

Biomicroscopy
(Slit Lamp Examination)

PURPOSE
To provide a highly magnified view of the eye.

The slit lamp permits the diagnosis and treatment of lesions in various areas of the eye such as the cornea, iris, and lens, and, with appropriate attachments, the retina and posterior vitreous.

TIME
Ten to 15 minutes.

LOCATION
Treatment room or physician's office.

PERSONNEL
Physician.

ROOM AND EQUIPMENT
Darkened room; slit lamp (a microscope with a special light source mounted on an instrument table) (Fig. 3-1).

PREPARATION
Examination of certain areas of the eye, e.g., the retina, necessitates dilation (see section on pupil dilatation, page 55).

TECHNIQUE
The patient is seated on one side of the slit lamp table with his chin and head supported by appropriate extensions of the slit lamp frame. He is directed to look straight ahead without blinking.

The physician manipulates the light source and microscope to visualize the eye structures under examination. As part of this procedure he may also elect to do applanation tonometry (see page 62) or other special studies.

PATIENT SENSATIONS AND AFTERCARE
See section on pupil dilatation.

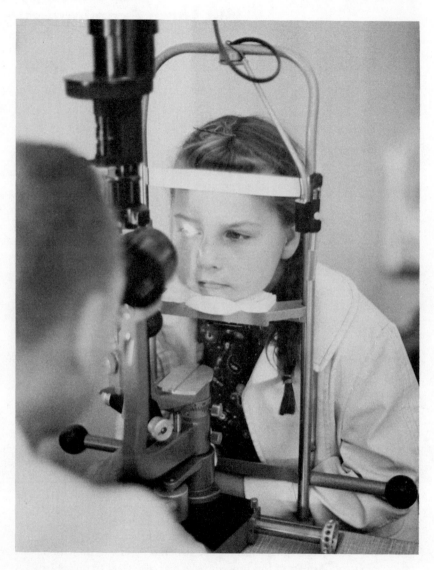

Figure 3-1. Patient being examined with slit lamp. (Courtesy Elizabeth Wilcox, Columbia-Presbyterian Medical Center, New York.)

Corneal Staining

PURPOSE Evaluation of the integrity of the corneal epithelium. Alterations in the epithelium may occur as a result of such insults as foreign bodies, burns, or abrasions.

TIME Five minutes. The time may be extended if irregularities are found; sketches of the eye with the location and general shape of the irregularities may be drawn, or further treatment may be instituted.

LOCATION Examining room or physician's office.

PERSONNEL Physician.

EQUIPMENT Fluorescein-impregnated paper strips.

PREPARATION None.

TECHNIQUE
1. The patient is seated and asked to stare straight ahead.
2. An anesthetic eye drop may be instilled if the physician anticipates that the nature of the lesion may make the examination painful.
3. The fluorescein paper strip is dampened with sterile saline solution and touched to the conjunctiva so that a thin film of dye spreads over the corneal surface.
4. Normal corneal tissue will not retain the dye. Any irregularity will be stained by the fluorescein.
5. The stained area of the cornea is usually sketched in on a drawing of the eye so that healing progress can be demonstrated.

PATIENT SENSATIONS As the anesthetic eye drops are instilled, the patient may have a mild burning sensation followed by a numb feeling similar to that experienced after the application of Novocain in the mouth.

AFTERCARE

1. The fluorescein dye stains the sclera a yellow orange color and is removed by the eye's normal cleansing mechanism.
2. If fluorescein drops onto the skin, it may easily be removed with clear water.
3. Approximately 30 minutes are required for the local anesthetic to dissipate. During this period of time extreme caution must be exercised to avoid inadvertent injury to the eyes. The patient's hands and any objects should be kept away from the eyes. If the patient must be outdoors, glasses should be worn to afford extra protection.

Tonometry

PURPOSE   Measurement of intraocular pressure by inward displacement or flattening of the cornea with a tonometer.
This test is used primarily to screen for and validate effective treatment of glaucoma.

TIME   Five to 10 minutes.

LOCATION   Examining room, bedside, or physician's office.

PERSONNEL   Physician.

EQUIPMENT   Schiøtz (Fig. 3-2) or applanation tonometer, anesthetic eye drops, and fluorescein-impregnated paper strips.

PREPARATION   None.

TECHNIQUE   A. Indentation tonometry (Schiøtz technique)
1. The patient must be positioned so that his head is firmly supported and his eyes are fully open. This is best achieved by either placing the patient supine

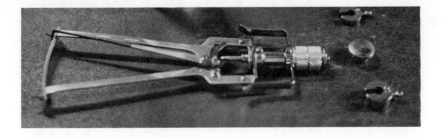

Figure 3-2. Schiøtz tonometer for measuring intraocular pressure. (Courtesy Lucy B. Lazzopina, Columbia-Presbyterian Medical Center, New York.)

in bed or seating him in an examining chair with a head support similar to that used by a dentist.

2. An anesthetic solution is instilled into both eyes.
3. The patient is asked to stare at a spot directly in his line of vision.
4. The eyelids are held apart and the tonometer is placed over the cornea. The central part of the tonometer contains a plunger which causes inward displacement of the cornea. The section coming in contact with the cornea resembles a contact lens in size and shape. The degree to which the cornea is displaced is recorded on the tonometer. The actual intraocular pressure is determined by a chart which converts the scale reading into millimeters of mercury. Normal intraocular pressure ranges from 15 to 25 mm of mercury.
5. This same maneuver is repeated on the other eye.

B. Applanation tonometry
1. The patient is seated in front of the slit lamp.
2. Anesthetic eye drops are instilled, and a fluorescein-impregnated paper strip is touched to the cornea.
3. The patient leans forward, resting his chin and fore-head on the slit lamp supports.
4. A plastic cone-shaped device containing two prisms and attached to the slit lamp is touched to the cornea.
5. A blue light projected through the prism device onto the cornea causes the dye to fluoresce.
6. The knobs on the tonometer are turned, gradually flattening the cornea. When the two prisms within the cone are aligned, intraocular pressure is read from a dial on the tonometer. The fluorescein and blue light enable the physician to visualize the prism pattern clearly.

PATIENT SENSATIONS

1. As the anesthetic eye drops are instilled and the fluo-rescein paper strip is applied, the patient may have a mild burning sensation followed by a numb feeling similar to that experienced after the application of Novocain in the mouth.
2. As the cornea is anesthetized before the procedure, no pain should be experienced.

3. The patient may experience unexpressed fear at the thought of an object being placed on the eye. Assurance should be given that the tonometer will be supported at all times by the physician or the slit lamp and that the eye will not be damaged by the instrument.

AFTERCARE

1. Approximately 30 minutes are required for the local anesthetic to wear off. During this period extreme caution must be exercised to avoid inadvertent injury to the eyes. The patient's hands and other objects should be kept away from the eyes. If the patient must be outdoors, glasses should be worn to afford extra protection.
2. The fluorescein dye which stains the sclera a yellow orange color is removed by the eye's normal cleansing mechanism.
3. If the fluorescein drips onto the skin, it may easily be removed with clear water.

Binocular Indirect Ophthalmoscopy

PURPOSE   Stereoscopic visualization of the posterior portion of the eye exclusive of the orbit.

This procedure permits examination of a wider angle of the eye than is possible with an ordinary ophthalmoscope.

TIME   Fifteen to 30 minutes.

LOCATION   Bedside, examining room, or physician's office.

PERSONNEL   Physician.

EQUIPMENT   Mydriatic-cycloplegic eye drops, convex lens, and binocular indirect ophthalmoscope. The ophthalmoscope, driven by a transformer or battery, is placed on the physician's head like a miner's helmet and includes the light source (Fig. 3-3).

PREPARATION   Dilation of both eyes to overcome the constrictive effect of the bright light on the pupils (see section on pupil dilation, page 55).

TECHNIQUE   The patient is seated in an examining chair with a head support similar to that used by a dentist. The physician, using the indirect ophthalmoscope and convex lens, examines each eye separately, instructing the patient to focus and maintain his gaze in various directions as each segment of the posterior eye is examined. Cooperation of the patient in following directions is essential to a complete examination. The physician may use one hand to hold open the eye being examined, while using the other to hold the convex lens over the eye. The convex lens projects the image seen through the indirect ophthalmoscope.

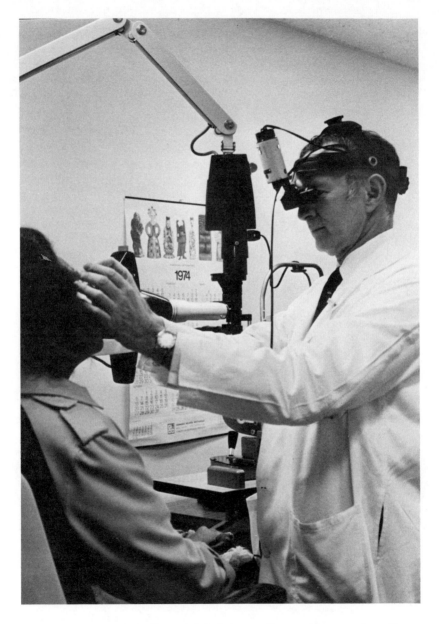

Figure 3-3.   Binocular indirect ophthalmoscope in use.   (Courtesy Lucy B. Lazzopina, Columbia-Presbyterian Medical Center, New York.)

**PATIENT
SENSATIONS
AND
AFTERCARE**

1. Postdilatation care should be instituted (see section on pupil dilatation).
2. When the procedure is performed on a patient who has recently undergone eye surgery, a mild analgesic may be required afterward, as movement of the eye postoperatively can cause discomfort.

Fluorescein Angiography

PURPOSE
Evaluation of the retinal and choroidal circulation of the eye.

This study is especially helpful in documenting hemorrhagic macular degeneration, diabetic neovascularization, diabetic retinopathy, and aneurysms.

TIME
Up to 1 hour.

LOCATION
Examining room or physician's office.

PERSONNEL
Physician and assistant.

EQUIPMENT
Sterile fluorescein dye for intravenous injection, mydriatic-cycloplegic eye drops, binocular indirect ophthalmoscope and fundus camera. The fundus camera resembles a 35-mm camera. It is mounted on an instrument table with a built-in light source.

PREPARATION
The pupil is dilated prior to injection of the dye to allow visualization of the retina (see section on pupil dilatation, page 55).

TECHNIQUE
1. The patient is seated in an examining chair, or on a stool in front of the fundus camera if pictures are desired. His chin and forehead are immobilized in a frame to permit proper focusing of the photographs.
2. Fluorescein dye is rapidly injected into the antecubital vein.
3. The circulation of the eye is then examined with the indirect ophthalmoscope (see section on binocular indirect ophthalmoscopy, page 64).
4. A series of pictures delineating retinal and choroidal circulation may be taken with the fundus camera starting

within seconds after the dye injection. Pictures may be taken for a period of 1 hour since certain abnormalities are not immediately manifest.

PATIENT SENSATIONS

1. See section on pupil dilatation.
2. The patient will experience the discomfort associated with venipuncture.
3. Occasionally nausea may be experienced immediately after the injection of fluorescein. This sensation is transitory.
4. Syncope is a possibility.

AFTERCARE

1. See section on pupil dilatation.
2. Patients should be advised that for approximately 24 hours after this examination their urine will be reddish in color.

Bibliography

Lyle, T. K., Cross, A. G., and Cook, C. A. G. *May and Worth's Manual of Diseases of the Eye* (13th ed.). Philadelphia: Davis, 1968.

Moses, R. A. *Adler's Physiology of the Eye: Clinical Application* (5th ed.). St. Louis: Mosby, 1970.

Scheie, H. G., and Albert, D. M. *Adler's Textbook of Ophthalmology* (8th ed.). Philadelphia: Saunders, 1969.

Vaughan, D., Asbury, T., and Cook, R. *General Ophthalmology* (6th ed.). Los Altos, Calif.: Lange, 1971.

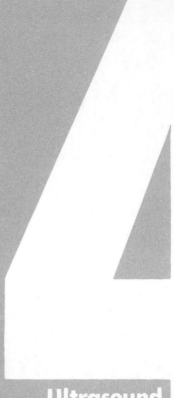

Ultrasound Procedures*

*N.B.: To ensure adequate understanding of the terminology, read the discussion on the purpose of ultrasonography (page 73) before proceeding.

Ultrasonography

PURPOSE   Utilization of ultrasound for imaging of soft tissues.

The tissues most commonly studied are the kidneys, liver, spleen, pancreas, gallbladder, thyroid, heart, eye, female reproductive organs, lymph nodes, and aorta.

Ultrasound is very high frequency, inaudible, vibratory sound waves. The sound waves are generated by a transducer consisting of a special vibrating crystal. The same transducer receives the returning echoes. The echo is produced when a sound wave passes through the junction of two tissues of differing densities. This junction is called an interface.

Ultrasound echoes can be displayed by A-mode (amplitude modulation) or B-mode (brightness modulation) on an oscilloscope. B-mode displays can be utilized differently according to the information sought. One of the modifications is the B-scan, in which scanning apparatus is added to the standard ultrasound equipment. This combination produces a two-dimensional view shown on the oscilloscope as a pattern of dots depicting an anatomically accurate cross-section through an organ at a given instant in time. An example of a B-scan ultrasonogram is shown in Figure 4-1.

TIME   Fifteen to 30 minutes.

LOCATION   Ultrasonography diagnostic suite. These procedures may sometimes be done at the bedside using a portable machine.

PERSONNEL   Physician and technician.

EQUIPMENT   Transducer, ultrasound scanner (scanning apparatus which holds the transducer and records its position at all times, and thus the position and depth of each echo source), amplifier, oscilloscope on which the echo pattern is displayed, and Polaroid camera for photographing significant oscilloscope displays.

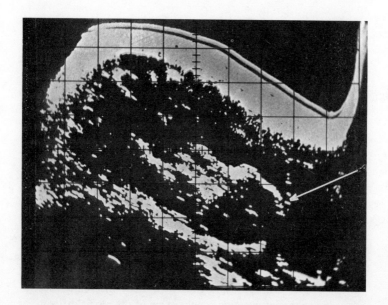

Figure 4-1. B-scan ultrasonogram of the placenta showing normal gestation at 20 weeks. Circular structure is fetal head. (Courtesy Donald L. King, M.D., Department of Radiology, Columbia-Presbyterian Medical Center, New York.)

PREPARATION 1. The patient must be able to lie still for the duration of the test. Any condition that precludes this should receive appropriate attention prior to the examination. Sedation may be necessary if the patient is unable to cooperate.

2. For obstetrical and gynecological ultrasonography, the patient is asked to drink three to four glasses of water immediately prior to the examination and not to empty her bladder until its completion. A full bladder enhances transmission of sound waves and improves visualization of pelvic organs.

3. Fasting is sometimes required before gallbladder ultrasonography.

4. Ultrasonography should be performed prior to any barium study, as ultrasound transmission is impeded by barium.

TECHNIQUE
1. The patient is usually placed in a supine or prone position depending on the organ under investigation.
2. Insulating gel is applied to the transducer and to the area under study to provide airtight contact. Air hinders ultrasound transmission.
3. With the transducer in contact with the skin, it is passed smoothly back and forth at various angles and in different directions. The display on the oscilloscope is observed closely and photographs are taken when significant patterns appear (Fig. 4-2).

PATIENT SENSATIONS
1. This is a painless, harmless, noninvasive procedure and easily tolerated by the patient.

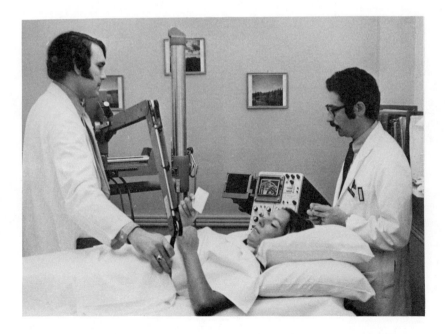

Figure 4-2. Patient undergoing abdominal ultrasonography. Photograph shows scanning apparatus, transducer held in position on abdomen, and oscilloscope with Polaroid camera swung away from screen. (Courtesy Beth Israel Hospital, Boston, Mass.)

2. As the transducer is moved back and forth, it produces a rubbing sensation. In the effort to maintain complete contact with the skin, enough pressure may be exerted to cause the patient minimal discomfort. However, many patients experience the pressure as a comfortable massage.

AFTERCARE   None.

Echocardiography

PURPOSE   To record motion of the heart valves and walls.

This study is performed to evaluate a suspected pericardial effusion, mitral stenosis, aortic regurgitation, and other abnormalities.

Echocardiography should not be confused with ultrasonography of the heart. An echocardiogram is a record of heart motion, while an ultrasonogram is an anatomical picture of the heart.

Echocardiography is an example of another modification of B-mode display. The echo pattern is displayed as a wave in which the vertical dimension measures depth inward from the chest wall, and the horizontal dimension represents time (time-motion display or M-mode). The width between two wave peaks is equivalent to one heart cycle (Fig. 4-3).

TIME   Fifteen to 30 minutes.

LOCATION   Ultrasonography diagnostic suite or bedside.

PERSONNEL   Physician or technician.

EQUIPMENT   Transducer, amplifier, display oscilloscope, and recording device (Polaroid camera or strip chart recorder).

PREPARATION   The ability to lie quietly during the test is a prerequisite for an accurate examination.

TECHNIQUE
1. The patient is placed in a supine position on the examining table.
2. A water-soluble gel is applied to the skin of the chest wall and to the end of the transducer.

Figure 4-3. Echocardiogram showing normal mitral valve function. (Courtesy Donald L. King, M.D., Department of Radiology, Columbia-Presbyterian Medical Center, New York.)

3. The examiner places the transducer on the chest wall so that it is in complete contact, and smoothly passes it back and forth over the area of the heart at various angles and in different directions. The oscilloscope or strip chart is carefully observed. The patient may be assisted to modify his position according to what is seen.
4. When adequate information has been obtained, the examination is concluded and the gel removed from the patient's skin.

PATIENT SENSATIONS   The patient will feel pressure and a rubbing sensation as the transducer is moved about the chest wall.

AFTERCARE   None.

Echoencephalography

PURPOSE   To measure the position of the midline structures of the brain.

The results of echoencephalography are viewed on an oscilloscope using an A-mode display. Figure 4-4 shows a representative display. The echoes produce spikes which indicate the depth of echo sources (interfaces) in the brain.

TIME   Ten to 15 minutes.

LOCATION   Ultrasonography diagnostic suite or bedside.

PERSONNEL   Physician and technician.

EQUIPMENT   Transducers, amplifier, display oscilloscope, and Polaroid camera.

PREPARATION   None.

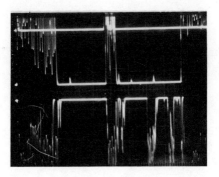

Figure 4-4. Normal echoencephalogram. (Courtesy Donald L. King, M.D., Department of Radiology, Columbia-Presbyterian Medical Center, New York.)

TECHNIQUE

1. The patient is either seated or placed in a supine position and must remain still until the procedure is concluded.
2. A water-soluble gel is applied to the patient's skull immediately above both ears to establish airtight contact with the transducers.
3. Two transducers are placed, one on either side of the head in the temporoparietal region above the ear. A series of spikes of varying heights is displayed on the oscilloscope and represents the diameter of the head.

   A single transducer is then placed first above one ear, then the other, and echoes from within the brain are recorded to determine the position of the midline structures. A difference in alignment of the midline echoes of 2.5 mm or greater is indicative of an abnormal shift in the midline structures and suggests the presence of a space-occupying lesion. Significant oscilloscopic displays are photographed.
4. After sufficient information has been obtained, the examination is concluded and the gel removed from the patient's head.

PATIENT SENSATIONS

There will be a sensation of gentle pressure and rubbing as the transducer is moved in different directions.

AFTERCARE

None.

Eye Ultrasonography

PURPOSE To determine the presence and nature of structural or
functional abnormalities of the eye.
Since this procedure does not depend on direct visualization,
it is particularly useful when an opacity prevents visualization of structures lying behind it.

TIME Five to 30 minutes, depending on whether an abnormality
is being identified or confirmed.

PERSONNEL Physician and technician.

LOCATION Ultrasonography diagnostic room.

**ROOM AND
EQUIPMENT** Darkened room, transducer, ultrasound scanner, amplifier,
two oscilloscopes for A- and B-mode displays, Polaroid
camera, double-ring apparatus of adjustable height which
supports a water bath, disposable OR drapes, collodion,
warm sterile saline solution, eyelid retractor, anesthetic and
mydriatic-cycloplegic eye drops, and examining table.

PREPARATION None unless dilatation is necessary for proper imaging of the
lens and anterior chamber (refer to pupil dilatation pro-
cedure, page 55). The examination may be performed on
an outpatient basis.

TECHNIQUE One of the crucial factors in eye ultrasonography is achieving
an airtight seal between the eye and the transducer. Several
methods are in use and there is continuous effort to find a
simpler, universally effective means of achieving this. Although the method described here is one of several in current
use for B-mode scanning, both A- and B-mode displays may
be obtained.

1. With the patient lying supine on the examining table, collodion is applied around the orbit of the eye and a disposable, waterproof, fenestrated OR drape is carefully applied, leaving the eye exposed. The outside ring of the double-ring apparatus is swung into position above the patient's eye and the edges of the drape are brought up through the ring and folded back over its edge. The second ring is fitted snugly over the towel-draped inner ring in the manner in which material is secured by an embroidery hoop. This forms a watertight cone-shaped structure known as a water bath. It widens out from the patient's exposed eye to the supporting ring structure (Fig. 4-5).
2. An anesthetic drop is instilled in the eye. If dilatation is necessary, mydriatic-cycloplegic drops are also instilled.

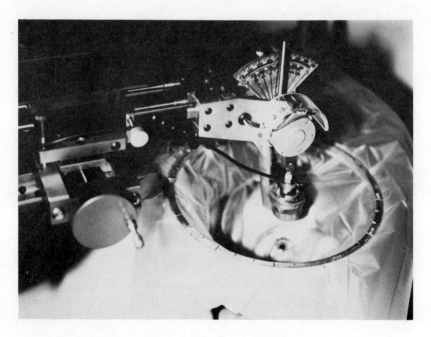

Figure 4-5. Equipment for eye ultrasonography showing scanning arm with transducer positioned over eye and water bath. (Courtesy D. Jackson Coleman, M.D., Edward S. Harkness Eye Institute, Columbia-Presbyterian Medical Center, New York.)

3. The patient is asked to look first down, then up, and not to blink as the eyelid retractor is applied. Because of the anesthetic eye drop, the patient is usually unaware of placement of the retractor.
4. Warm sterile saline solution is poured gently into the water bath until the eye is submerged. This serves as a seal, preventing any air from coming between the eye and the transducer. Fluid transmits sound waves; air or gas interferes with their transmission.
5. The transducer is then partially immersed in the water bath and passed back and forth over the eye at various angles. As the transducer is moved about, the patient is asked to look in different directions. This allows different segments and planes of the eye to be examined. When significant structural patterns appear on the oscilloscope, photographs are taken.
6. At the completion of the examination the retractor is removed. The patient is instructed to close his eye and the water bath is drained through a puncture made in the drape. The drape is then removed and the area around the eye dried with tissues.
7. If both eyes are to be examined, the procedure is repeated for the other eye.

If only A-mode display is desired, the method is not as involved. The patient usually sits in a chair in front of the examiner. A local anesthetic eye drop is instilled, followed by saline solution or methylcellulose drops; the latter two provide a film of fluid contact. The transducer is placed directly on the eye or lids and manually moved in different directions across the eye. The oscilloscope display is observed and appropriate photographs taken.

PATIENT SENSATIONS

1. Persons who have had an eye ultrasonogram describe the sensation of the eye's being submerged in fluid as "eerie" or "weird," but not painful. It can be compared to swimming under water with open eyes, but because of the anesthetic eye drop, without discomfort or pain.
2. The patient may experience sympathetic tearing of the other eye.

AFTERCARE
1. The topical anesthetic wears off within 20 to 30 minutes of administration. Thus its effect is over shortly after the procedure. However, the patient should be instructed to avoid rubbing his eyes and to wear glasses if going outdoors immediately. This will protect the eye from injury.
2. If dilatation has been done, the patient should receive appropriate instructions (see pupil dilatation procedure).
3. When the collodion dries, it will usually flake off the skin easily. If it does not, cold cream or soap and water will remove it completely. Removal should not be attempted until the topical anesthetic has worn off.

Bibliography

Coleman, D. J.   Reliability of ocular and orbital diagnosis with B-scan ultrasound: 1. Ocular diagnosis. *Am. J. Ophthalmol.* 73:501, 1972.

Coleman, D. J.   Reliability of ocular and orbital diagnosis with B-scan ultrasound: 2. Orbital diagnosis. *Am. J. Ophthalmol.* 74:704, 1972.

Cubberly, M. G.   Photography of ultrasound scans in diagnostic ophthalmology. *J. Biol. Photogr. Assoc.* 41:39, 1973.

Doust, B. D.   Role of ultrasound in obstetrics and gynecology. *Hosp. Prac.* 8:143, 1973.

Ellis, K., and King, D. L.   Pericarditis and pericardial effusion: Radiologic and echocardiographic diagnosis. *Radiol. Clin. North Am.* 11:393, 1973.

Feigenbaum, H.   *Echocardiography.* Philadelphia: Lea & Febiger, 1972.

King, D. L.   Cardiac ultrasonography. *Circulation* 47:843, 1973.

King, D. L.   Placental ultrasonography. *J. Clin. Ultrasound* 1:21, 1973.

Leopold, G. R., and Asher, G. R.   Ultrasound in obstetrics and gynecology. *Radiol. Clin. North Am.* 12:127, 1974.

Leopold, G. R., and Sokoloff, J.   Ultrasonic scanning in the diagnosis of biliary disease. *Surg. Clin. North Am.* 53:1043, 1973.

Seat, S. G.   B-scan abdominal and retroperitoneal echography. Teaching file, Department of Radiology, Scripps Clinic and Research Foundation, La Jolla, Calif. Revised February 1974.

Wells, P. N. T. (Ed.).   *Ultrasonics in Clinical Diagnosis.* Baltimore: Williams & Wilkins, 1972.

5

Biliary System and Gastrointestinal Tract

Oral Cholecystography

PURPOSE   Roentgenographic visualization of the gallbladder.

TIME   The total time of the procedure is about 30 to 45 minutes. Much of this time is spent waiting while the films are processed and examined. This continuous inspection guides the remainder of the procedure.

LOCATION   Radiology department.

PERSONNEL   Technician.

EQUIPMENT   Conventional x-ray table with overhead apparatus.

PREPARATION   1. Unless contraindicated because of pain, normal fat intake should be maintained for several days prior to oral cholecystography in order to empty the bile from the gallbladder. If this is not possible, at least the midday meal on the day preceding the examination should contain a normal amount of fat.

2. A fat-free meal is eaten the evening prior to the examination. Outpatients should be instructed that only lean meats, fruits, vegetables, bread, and coffee or tea are permitted. Eggs, butter, milk, salad oils, and fatty meats should be excluded. This fat-free meal prevents gallbladder contraction and thus permits accumulation of the contrast material within it.

3. The patient remains fasting except for water and tea or coffee (without cream or milk) from 10:00 P.M. the evening prior to the procedure until its completion. This permits gallbladder concentration of the contrast material with the bile.

4. The contrast material is taken early in the evening prior to the procedure. Although other contrast media are

available, iopanoic acid U.S.P. (Telepaque tablets) is commonly used. Six 500-mg tablets should be taken at 5-minute intervals to minimize nausea. It is important that the schedule specified by the institution be adhered to strictly to provide sufficient time for adequate absorption of the contrast material.

5. Oral cholecystography precedes any barium study.

TECHNIQUE

1. Initial films are obtained to determine the position of the gallbladder and to ensure that it has opacified.
2. If the gallbladder is visualized on the preliminary films, the patient is given a fatty meal.
3. Contraction of the gallbladder in response to the fat stimulus requires 15 to 20 minutes. After gallbladder contraction, additional overhead films are exposed.
4. If stones are clearly detected on the preliminary films, no fat is administered and the procedure is terminated.
5. In some instances, particularly when the initial films demonstrate indeterminate findings, fluoroscopy with spot filming is done.

PATIENT SENSATIONS

1. There is no pain or discomfort associated with the procedure itself.
2. Although many patients experience no side-effects from the Telepaque tablets, some do have nausea, vomiting, diarrhea, and dysuria. If any of the GI symptoms are severe, the radiology department should be informed. If on the initial films the gallbladder fails to opacify, poor absorption of the contrast material, rather than underlying gallbladder disease, may be considered as causal.

AFTERCARE

1. No special care is required if the entire procedure has been performed.
2. If the gallbladder was not visualized or only poorly visualized, a repeat dose of 3 gm of Telepaque is given that evening and the procedure is repeated the following day. Although failure of opacification may be indicative of gallbladder disease, it may also result from inadequate

absorption of the contrast material. It should be emphasized to the patient that repetition of the procedure is not due to a technical error but is rather a necessary part of the process.

Intravenous Cholangiography (IVC)

PURPOSE   Roentgenographic visualization of the biliary ducts and gallbladder, if present.

This procedure is performed when the gallbladder has not been visualized during oral cholecystography or when biliary symptoms occur in a patient who has had a cholecystectomy.

TIME   Two to 4 hours. Since each film is processed and inspected immediately, there may be indications either for terminating the procedure before this time or for extending it.

LOCATION   Radiology department.

PERSONNEL   Radiologist to inject the contrast material; technician to take the films.

EQUIPMENT   X-ray table with overhead apparatus, and tomographic equipment.

PREPARATION   1. In some hospitals, a fatty diet is eaten for the two days preceding the test to empty the gallbladder.
2. A strong cathartic is taken the afternoon before the procedure, as a bowel free of gas and feces permits clearer visualization.
3. The patient remains fasting from midnight prior to the procedure until after its completion. Fat-free liquids are permitted, however, and their consumption should be encouraged. Side-effects are minimized when the patient is well hydrated.
4. Intravenous cholangiography precedes any barium study.

TECHNIQUE   1. With the patient prone and his right side elevated, a scout film* is taken.

*An x-ray film exposed before any contrast material is injected.

2. A small amount of the contrast material, Cholografin meglumine (meglumine iodipamide injection U.S.P.) is given intravenously. If no hypersensitivity reaction occurs within 3 minutes, the remainder is given slowly, either directly into the vein or by infusion. Side-effects are minimized by slow injection.

3. Usually a series of films is taken starting 15 to 20 minutes after the injection and at intervals of 20 minutes thereafter until maximum visualization of the biliary ducts occurs, usually within 30 to 60 minutes. If the gallbladder and the cystic duct are patent, gallbladder opacification will occur in 1 to 2 hours. If there is an obstruction in any part of the biliary system, opacification will be delayed and the procedure extended accordingly.

4. Tomographic cuts* are routinely obtained, particularly when extraneous shadows do not permit adequate visualization.

PATIENT SENSATIONS

1. Many patients experience some side-effects from the Cholografin. Minor symptoms include nausea, vomiting, flushing, and urticaria. More severe and potentially fatal reactions include anaphylaxis and cardiovascular collapse. The patient should report *any* untoward sensation so that corrective measures may be instituted.

2. While the tomographic cuts are being taken, the patient must retain the same posture. This is an obvious source of discomfort, and he should be assured that foam wedges will be used to assist him in maintaining his position and that the personnel of the radiology department will be available should further assistance be necessary. He will be required to remain on the x-ray

---

*Tomograms, laminagrams, planigrams, or body section roetgenograms: By adjusting the x-ray equipment so that there is simultaneous movement of the x-ray tube and the film in opposite directions about a specific plane, all structures are blurred out, leaving only a selected layer of an organ in clear view. Films obtained in this manner are often called tomographic cuts.

The two x-ray tubes which make up tomographic equipment are suspended over the x-ray table. When the cuts are being made, these swing rapidly and abruptly in converging and then diverging paths above the patient. This rapid swooping may frighten the patient if he is not forewarned.

table between exposures only during the tomographic study.

AFTERCARE   If untoward reactions occur as a result of the contrast material, the patient or staff will be informed of any special instructions.

Postoperative Cholangiography
(T-tube Cholangiography)

PURPOSE
Roentgenographic visualization of the biliary ducts.
This study is routinely performed approximately 7 to 10 days after surgery and prior to T-tube removal to assess the patency of the ductal system and to look for residual calculi.

TIME
Fifteen minutes.

LOCATION
Radiology department.

PERSONNEL
Radiologist and technician.

EQUIPMENT
X-ray table and fluoroscopy unit.

PREPARATION
In some institutions the T-tube is drained by gravity for 24 hours prior to the procedure to fill it with bile. This ensures the absence of air bubbles which may simulate calculi on the x-ray film.

TECHNIQUE
The patient is placed in a supine position on the x-ray table. Under fluoroscopic guidance the contrast material is injected directly into the T-tube. Spot films are obtained throughout the procedure depending on what is seen fluoroscopically.

PATIENT SENSATIONS
Although no pain is associated with T-tube cholangiography, some patients may experience a feeling of fullness in the right upper quadrant as the contrast material is injected.

AFTERCARE
If the ducts are found to be free of abnormalities, the T-tube is removed.

Percutaneous Transhepatic Cholangiography

PURPOSE   Roentgenographic visualization of the biliary ducts.

This procedure is performed primarily to differentiate between obstructive and nonobstructive jaundice. Conventional cholangiography often fails to outline the biliary system in jaundiced patients. If percutaneous transhepatic cholangiography shows obstruction, surgery is scheduled to follow immediately.

TIME   Thirty minutes.

LOCATION   Radiology department.

PERSONNEL   Radiologist and technician.

EQUIPMENT   Tilting x-ray table and fluoroscopy unit.

TECHNIQUE
1. The patient is placed in a supine position on the x-ray table. The skin over the liver is cleansed with an antiseptic solution and sterilely draped. The skin, intervening tissues, and liver capsule are then infiltrated with a local anesthetic.
2. Under fluoroscopic guidance the liver is punctured with a long needle. The patient is instructed to hold his breath on expiration as the needle enters the liver.
3. The needle is directed into a biliary duct and as much bile as possible is aspirated. If a biliary duct is not entered, the needle is redirected until one is identified. Usually the procedure is terminated if a duct cannot be found after several attempts. Failure to locate a duct is suggestive of hepatocellular disease, as the ducts are usually dilated in obstructive disease and therefore easily located.

4. The examination is carried out with the table horizontal and upright or semiupright and the patient positioned in various degrees of obliquity.
5. The contrast material is injected into the identified duct after aspiration of bile. Opacification of the biliary ducts is observed fluoroscopically and spot films are taken.
6. At the conclusion of the fluoroscopic examination the needle is withdrawn and routine overhead radiographs are exposed.

PREPARATION
1. Clotting mechanisms are evaluated prior to the procedure. Any deviations must be corrected before its performance.
2. The patient remains fasting before the procedure.
3. Premedication is administered in order to minimize anxiety and thus elicit the greatest degree of cooperation.

PATIENT SENSATIONS
1. When the local anesthetic is administered, the patient will experience a stinging sensation as the skin is injected and transitory pain as the liver capsule is entered.
2. Because the area is anesthetized, the patient should experience no pain but may feel pressure from the liver puncture.
3. If the volume of contrast medium is excessive, the patient will experience a sensation of epigastric fullness with pain in the back or right upper quadrant. The pain ceases as soon as the injection has been completed.
4. The patient should be assured that he will be adequately secured to the table and therefore should not be frightened when it is tilted.

AFTERCARE
1. If the results confirm the necessity for surgery, it is usually performed within several hours after the procedure.
2. If surgery is not indicated, the patient must be observed for hemorrhage secondary to inadvertent puncture of a blood vessel or for bile peritonitis from leakage of bile into the peritoneal cavity, or both.

Barium Enema

PURPOSE Roentgenographic visualization of the entire large intestine.

TIME Thirty to 45 minutes.

LOCATION Radiology department.

PERSONNEL Radiologist and technician.

EQUIPMENT Fluoroscopy unit and x-ray table with overhead apparatus.

TECHNIQUE With the patient in a lateral recumbent position, a rectal catheter is inserted. Under fluoroscopic guidance the barium mixture is instilled by means of gravity into the large intestine. Throughout the procedure the barium is administered slowly and incrementally, and the patient is rotated into various positions in order to visualize all flexures and loops of the colon. Spot films are taken depending on what is observed fluoroscopically.

Some form of compression is applied intermittently to the abdomen to separate overlying loops of bowel and to detect small lesions (Fig. 5-1). After complete filling of the colon several overhead films are exposed. The patient is then assisted to the bathroom to expel the barium. After evacuation overhead films are taken to detect mucosal abnormalities.

Should polyps be suspected or bleeding have occurred in a patient with no hemorrhoids and negative findings on the barium enema study, an air contrast study is performed. Although some institutions do this as a separate procedure, others perform it immediately after the routine barium enema. After evacuation of the barium and while the mucosa still retains a thin coating of it, the colon is distended with air and further filming is done.

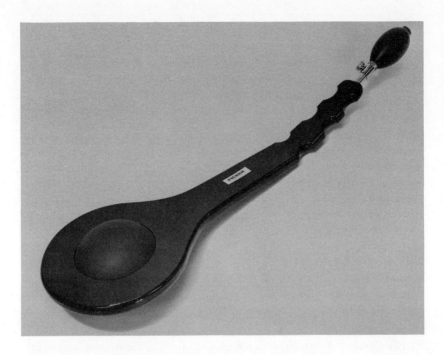

Figure 5-1. Pneumatic compression paddle. (Courtesy Picker Corporation, Cleveland, Ohio.)

PATIENT **1.** A barium enema is an extremely fatiguing, often difficult
SENSATIONS   procedure. In addition, many patients find it embarrass-
               ing, particularly if they are unable to retain the barium
               and expel it around the tube, or are unable to reach the
               bathroom before evacuating. It is important to anticipate
               this aspect of the examination, as patients often find it
               difficult to verbalize fears of embarrassment. By stating
               this feeling for them, much anxiety may be dissipated.
2. A feeling of fullness, cramping, and an urge to defecate
               accompany the instillation of barium.
3. If a double contrast study is done the patient will ex-
               perience moderate to severe cramps as the colon is distended
               with air.

PREPARATION **1.** Regardless of the method utilized, the objective of pre-
               paring for a barium enema is to cleanse the colon thoroughly

and completely. This is achieved by controlling diet and administering cathartics or enemas, or both. The presence of any gas or feces in the large intestine will make the quality and accuracy of the study questionable. Under these circumstances, the procedure may have to be repeated, causing great discomfort and incurring additional expense to the patient. Clearly, to be too lenient in enforcing the preparatory regimen is to do the patient a disservice.

2. If the barium enema is being administered through a colostomy, no cathartic is given. The usual preparation consists of a diet of clear liquids for 24 hours prior to the examination and a more vigorous irrigation the morning of the study.
3. A barium enema should precede an oral barium study if the latter is planned. Proctosigmoidoscopy, where indicated, should be done at least 1 day prior to a barium enema. At least 3 days and preferably a week should intervene between a colon biopsy and a barium enema.

AFTERCARE
1. An impaction may result from inspissation of barium in the large bowel. Therefore cleansing enemas or laxatives may be administered to rid the colon of the residual barium. In addition, fluid intake should be encouraged, unless contraindicated because of a coexisting medical problem, to accelerate rehydration. The extensive preparation required for a barium enema may in itself produce dehydration.
2. If enemas or cathartics are not part of the institutional protocol, the patient should be advised that his stool will be white for 24 to 72 hours following the examination.

Upper GI Series (UGIS) and Small Bowel Examination

PURPOSE

1. Upper GI series — roentgenographic visualization of the esophagus, stomach, and duodenum.
2. Small bowel examination — roentgenographic visualization of the small intestine up to and including the ileocecal junction. Although examination of the small bowel may be done as a separate procedure, it usually follows the upper GI series.

TIME

Upper GI series — 20 to 30 minutes.
Small bowel examination — 2 to 6 hours.

LOCATION

Radiology department.

PERSONNEL

Radiologist and technician.

EQUIPMENT

Fluoroscopy unit, overhead x-ray apparatus, and tilting x-ray table.

Some hospitals utilize remote-control equipment for GI fluoroscopy. The radiologist is in an adjacent room separated by a glass window through which he can see the patient and give verbal instructions. Otherwise, the radiologist remains in the same room as the patient.

PREPARATION

The patient remains fasting prior to the examination.

TECHNIQUE

A. Upper GI series
1. Unless the condition of the patient precludes it, the examination is begun with the table in a vertical position and the patient standing (Fig. 5-2).
2. The patient is given a cupful of barium. Throughout the procedure the radiologist will instruct him when to drink, how much to drink, and when to stop.

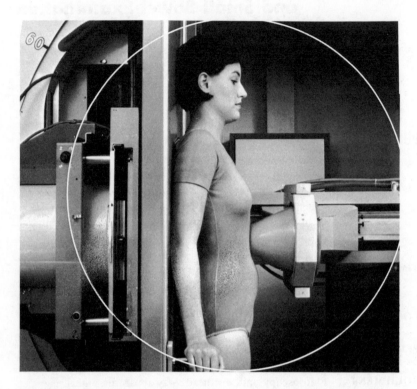

Figure 5-2. Tilting x-ray table in vertical position with patient standing. This particular model has compression device built into machine. (From Beranbaum, S. L., and Yaghmai, M. *Fluoroscopy and Radiology of the Gastrointestinal Tract.* Wilmington, Del. E. I. du Pont de Nemours and Co., 1967.)

3. Thorough opacification and visualization are achieved by tilting the table and by positioning the patient in various degrees of obliquity. The patient should be assured that he will be adequately secured to the table.

4. Spot films are taken throughout depending on what is visualized fluoroscopically.

5. Compression, either with a device made especially for that purpose or by the examiner's lead-gloved hand, may be

applied at any time throughout the procedure in order to spread the barium mixture and thus elicit maximal detail.

6. The examination is completed by exposing several overhead radiographs with the table in a horizontal position.

B. Small bowel examination
1. The patient drinks additional barium.
2. Overhead radiographs are exposed at 30-minute intervals unless previous filming has demonstrated rapid transit time. Each film is processed immediately to reveal how far the barium has advanced and determine whether additional fluoroscopy and spot filming are indicated.
3. The examination is terminated when the barium enters the cecum.
4. The patient usually remains in the radiology department throughout the examination. If the radiologist has determined that transit time will be delayed, the patient may be allowed to go to his room and return for the appointed films.

PATIENT SENSATIONS
1. There is no discomfort associated with the procedure.
2. The consistency of barium sulfate is similar to that of malted milk. Each radiology department attempts to disguise its chalklike taste with a more popular flavor such as strawberry or chocolate.
3. As the patient may need to remain in the radiology department for an extended period of time, he should be encouraged to bring some quiet diversional activity.

AFTERCARE
1. A cathartic may be administered to eliminate the barium.
2. If no cathartic is prescribed, the patient should be informed that his stool will be white for 24 to 72 hours after the test.

Esophagography (Barium Swallow)

PURPOSE   Roentgenographic visualization of the esophagus.

                           Although the esophagus is usually examined as an integral portion of a routine upper GI series, it may be examined independently when symptoms specifically related to it are present. Through particular maneuvers and positions, the structure, mucosal pattern, and swallowing function of the esophagus may be evaluated.

TIME   Twenty minutes.

LOCATION   Radiology department.

PERSONNEL   Radiologist and technician.

EQUIPMENT   Fluoroscopy unit and tilting x-ray table. As in the upper GI series, remote-control equipment may be used. In this case, the radiologist is in an adjacent room separated from the patient by a glass window. Otherwise, he remains in the same room with the patient.

PREPARATION None.

TECHNIQUE   The examination is begun with the patient in an upright position behind the fluoroscopic screen. After an initial fluoroscopic survey of the chest, the patient is instructed to swallow several mouthfuls of barium. Spot films are exposed with the patient rotated in various degrees of obliquity. The table is then tilted into a horizontal position and, with the patient supine and then prone on the table, these steps are repeated.

                           In addition, various maneuvers or techniques may be employed during the examination to elicit particular information. The following are examples:

1. To study the integrity of the cardioesophageal junction, the water siphonage test is performed. After the patient drinks a large amount of barium, the table is put in the Trendelenburg position and the patient is instructed to sip water continuously. Results are positive if there is a reflux of barium into the esophagus.

2. If a foreign body is suspected, the patient may be asked to swallow a cotton ball saturated with barium or a barium-filled gelatin capsule. This will localize the obstruction, to which the investigator may then direct attention.

3. To inspect the mucosal pattern of the esophagus, a double contrast study is done. This may be accomplished either by having the patient voluntarily swallow air with the barium or by having him sip barium through a straw with a pinhole in it.

4. To demonstrate a hiatal hernia or gastroesophageal reflux, intraabdominal pressure is raised by having the patient bear down or cough.

When cineradiographic apparatus is available, it may be employed during the procedure, particularly when the patient's main problem is a swallowing dysfunction. With use of this equipment, each phase of the process can be re-examined at a later time and in slow motion.

PATIENT SENSATIONS

1. There is no discomfort associated with esophagography.

2. The consistency of barium sulfate is similar to that of malted milk. Each radiology department attempts to disguise its chalklike taste with a more popular flavor such as strawberry or chocolate.

AFTERCARE

1. A cathartic may be administered to eliminate the barium.

2. If no cathartic is prescribed, the patient should be informed that his stool will be white for 24 to 72 hours after the test.

Hypotonic Duodenography

PURPOSE   Roentgenographic visualization of the duodenum and adjacent structures (Fig. 5-3).

                    This procedure is performed primarily to detect pancreatic disease.

TIME   Thirty minutes.

LOCATION   Radiology department.

PERSONNEL   Radiologist and technician.

EQUIPMENT   Tilting x-ray table, fluoroscopy unit, intestinal catheter, and anticholinergic medication.

TECHNIQUE   1. With the patient seated, a polyethylene catheter is passed through the nose into the stomach.

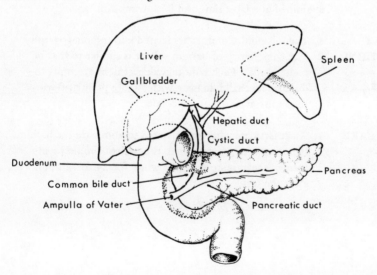

Figure 5-3.   Diagram of duodenum and adjacent structures.

2. The patient is then placed in a supine position and the catheter advanced under fluoroscopic guidance to the duodenum. The patient may be repositioned in order to accomplish this.
3. When the catheter is appropriately situated, an anticholinergic medication such as propantheline bromide (Pro-Banthīne) is administered intramuscularly or sometimes intravenously to produce duodenal atony. Approximately 5 minutes are required to produce this effect. More recently, glucagon has been used intravenously, as it has fewer side-effects.
4. Barium is then instilled through the catheter to visualize the configuration of the flaccid duodenal wall, which may be impinged on by adjacent pancreatic masses.
5. After spot films are obtained in various projections, some barium is withdrawn and replaced with air. Air contrast spot films are then exposed.
6. After completion of the filming, the catheter is removed.

PATIENT SENSATIONS

1. The patient may experience cramping pains as the air is introduced into the duodenum.
2. Many patients experience side-effects from the anticholinergic medication. These include tachycardia, dry mouth with thirst and difficulty in swallowing, blurred vision, and transient urinary retention, particularly in elderly men with prostatic hypertrophy. These symptoms may persist for several hours.

PREPARATION

1. This procedure may be contraindicated in those patients who cannot tolerate an anticholinergic medication because of the existence of other medical problems, such as glaucoma or severe heart disease with arrhythmias.
2. The patient remains fasting prior to the procedure.

AFTERCARE

After the procedure, voiding should be verified in men with prostatism. To obviate the possibility of urinary retention, men with this condition should void immediately before the procedure and restrict fluids for several hours after its completion.

Upper GI (UGI) Endoscopy

PURPOSE   Direct visualization of the esophagus, stomach, and duodenum.

Upper GI endoscopy is performed primarily as an adjunct to x-ray evaluation and as an emergency procedure in patients with acute upper GI bleeding.

TIME   Esophagoscopy — 15 minutes.
Gastroscopy — 15 to 30 minutes.
Duodenoscopy — 15 to 45 minutes.

Additional time will be required to achieve adequate local anesthesia and adequate relaxation.

LOCATION   Although usually performed in a special endoscopy suite with all the equipment readily available, this procedure can be done at the patient's bedside in an emergency situation, e.g., upper GI hemorrhage.

PERSONNEL   Gastroenterologist and nurse. As a second eyepiece can be mounted on the endoscopes for all three procedures, other physicians, nurses, and students may be present and can observe the findings simultaneously.

EQUIPMENT   Endoscope. Several types permit visualization of the esophagus, stomach, and duodenum with a single instrument (Fig. 5-4). Endoscopes designed specifically for each of the three areas are also available. The selection of instrument depends on the physician's preference and the particular information being sought. Although rigid instruments are still used in some institutions, only the newer, fiberoptic endoscopes will be described here.

Fiberoptic endoscopes are fully flexible instruments providing an undistorted image even when completely bent. The image is transmitted through a series of fiberglass bundles. Illumination is provided by an external light

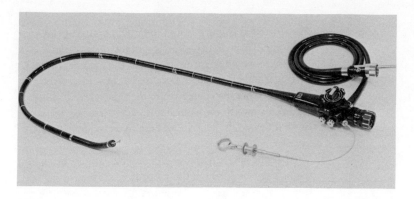

Figure 5-4. Gastrointestinal fiberoptic endoscope. (Courtesy Olympus Corporation of America, New Hyde Park, N.Y.)

source and conducted through a second set of fiber bundles (cold light source). The tip of the scope is controlled by the examiner and may be manipulated in all directions. There are channels for biopsy and air insufflation, attachments for suction, and an irrigating device to cleanse the distal lens. Cameras can be mounted on the proximal eyepiece to provide color photographs or movie films.

TECHNIQUE The patient's throat is anesthetized either by swabbing it with a local anesthetic or by having him gargle with the anesthetic. Five to 10 minutes are required to achieve adequate anesthesia. A sedative such as diazepam is then administered intravenously to relax the patient effectively without hindering his ability to cooperate during the examination.

When the patient is fully relaxed, he is placed in a left lateral recumbent position. The physician guides the endoscope to the hypopharynx, and by having the patient swallow, it is passed into the esophagus. The endoscope is further advanced to the anatomical area to be examined. Optimal visualization is achieved by air insufflation.

Biopsy specimens and brushings for cytological examination are taken when indicated.

PATIENT SENSATIONS 1. The local anesthesia will cause the patient's tongue and throat to feel swollen.

2. The patient may gag during the initial passage of the endoscope, but vomiting rarely occurs.

3. Although swallowing is unimpaired, the patient will feel as if he is unable to do so because of the local anesthesia. He is therefore instructed to let the saliva drain from the side of his mouth into a basin or paper tissues. A small suction device similar to that employed by dentists may be used.

4. The patient will experience a cramping pain as the endoscope is passed through the pylorus, and on air insufflation.

5. After completion of the examination, the patient may have a sore throat as a result of irritation by the endoscope. Lozenges may be prescribed to alleviate this discomfort.

6. If diazepam was given, the patient will have limited recall of the procedure owing to the amnesic action of the drug.

PREPARATION
1. Unless the procedure is performed on an emergency basis, all food and fluid as well as antacids are withheld to ensure optimum visualization and to prevent aspiration. If emergency endoscopy is performed, the stomach will be aspirated beforehand through a nasogastric tube.

2. Dentures are removed. Although a bite block is used during the procedure, inadvertent biting of the endoscope may damage either the dentures or the instrument.

3. If the procedure is to be done on an outpatient basis, the patient should be advised to come accompanied by someone who can assist him in returning home, especially if driving is necessary.

AFTERCARE
1. The hospitalized patient will return to his room after completion of the examination. Vital signs should be checked and side rails raised until the medication has worn off. The patient's mentation and gag reflex are evaluated before permitting food and fluid (which are generally withheld for 4 hours).

2. Any complaints of sharp, intense pain in the stomach or chest should be noted and reported immediately. Although perforation is a rare complication of upper GI endoscopy, these symptoms may be suggestive of it.

3. When the procedure is performed on an outpatient basis, the patient remains in the endoscopy suite until the sedation has worn off and the gag reflex returned. This may require as long as 3 hours.

Endoscopic Pancreatocholangiography

PURPOSE   Roentgenographic visualization of the pancreatic and biliary ducts by cannulation of the ampulla of Vater and injection of contrast material (see Fig. 5-3).

As this procedure is technically difficult and relatively new, its performance is currently limited to large medical centers.

TIME   Forty-five minutes to 2 1/2 hours.

LOCATION   Radiology department.

PERSONNEL   Gastroenterologist, radiologist, and technician.

EQUIPMENT   X-ray table, fluoroscopy unit, and duodenoscope (Fig. 5-5). For an explanation of the fiberoptic duodenoscope, refer to the section on upper GI endoscopy (pages 108–109).

PREPARATION   See the section on upper GI endoscopy.

TECHNIQUE   The application of a local anesthetic, the administration of sedation, and the insertion of the duodenoscope have been described under upper GI endoscopy and the reader is referred to that procedure.

An anticholinergic medication, such as propantheline bromide (Pro-Banthīne), is administered to produce duodenal atony. After passage of the fiberoptic duodenoscope, a cannula is inserted through the biopsy channel and positioned into the visualized ampulla of Vater. Contrast material is injected through the cannula, outlining the pancreatic and biliary ducts. Fluoroscopy, with spot films, is performed to visualize abnormalities of both ductal systems. The duodenoscope is then removed, the patient placed in a supine position, and additional overhead radiographs are obtained.

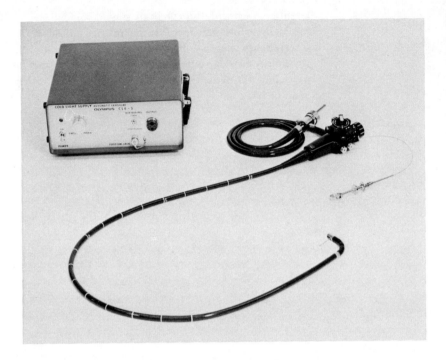

Figure 5-5. Fiberoptic duodenoscope with cold light source. (Courtesy Olympus Corporation of America, New Hyde Park, N.Y.)

PATIENT SENSATIONS   For sensations related to the application of anesthesia and the passage of the duodenoscope, refer to the section on upper GI endoscopy.

Many patients experience side-effects from the anticholinergic medication. These include tachycardia, dry mouth with thirst and difficulty in swallowing, blurred vision, and transient urinary retention, particularly in elderly men with prostatic hypertrophy. These symptoms may persist for several hours after the examination.

AFTERCARE   1. For care related to effects of anesthesia refer to the section on upper GI endoscopy.
2. After the procedure, voiding should be verified in men with prostatism. To obviate the possibility of urinary

retention, men with this condition should void immediately before the procedure and restrict fluids for several hours after its completion.

3. As cholecystitis or pancreatitis may be induced by this procedure, the patient should be observed for the development of fever and right upper quadrant pain.

Proctosigmoidoscopy

PURPOSE   Endoscopic visualization of the lower portion of the large intestine may take the form of sigmoidoscopy (rectum, rectosigmoid junction, and lower sigmoid), proctoscopy (rectum), or anoscopy (anus; this is usually included in a proctosigmoidoscopic examination). The three procedures differ only in the length of the endoscope employed and the specific portion of the mucosa that can be visualized.

A proctosigmoidoscopic examination may be performed on any patient with symptoms specifically related to the large intestine such as a change in bowel habits or bloody stool. It is also an integral feature of a complete physical examination in patients over 45 years of age to detect cancer.

TIME   Ten minutes.

LOCATION   Treatment room, endoscopy suite, or physician's office.

PERSONNEL   Physician and assistant.

EQUIPMENT   Rigid endoscope with light source (Fig. 5-6), anoscope, suction, air insufflator, and biopsy forceps.

PREPARATION   Colonic preparation usually consists of some form of enema or a stimulatory suppository.

TECHNIQUE   The patient assumes a knee-chest (Fig. 5-7) or left lateral recumbent position on the examination table. A tilt table is available which can be mechanically adjusted to the contours of the knee-chest position, thereby making that position easier to assume and maintain.

An initial digital rectal examination is performed to dilate the sphincter and to ascertain that no major obstruc-

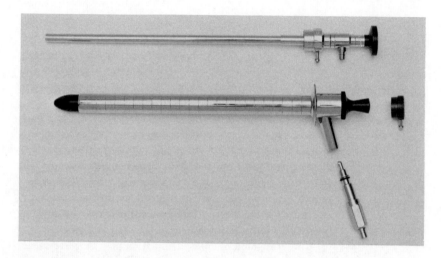

Figure 5-6. Proctosigmoidoscope with light attachment and obturator. (Courtesy American Cystoscope Makers, Inc., Stamford, Conn.)

tion to the endoscope exists. The endoscope is then gradually inserted to its full length if this can be accomplished without great discomfort. As it is slowly withdrawn, all areas of the intestinal mucosa are examined. Air is introduced through the endoscope to separate the mucosal folds and thus obtain maximal visualization. If suspect tissue is seen at any point, a biopsy specimen may be obtained; some polyps may also be excised.

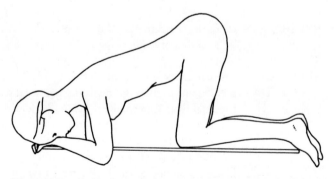

Figure 5-7. Knee-chest position for proctosigmoidoscopy.

PATIENT SENSATIONS

During the initial digital examination and the passage of the endoscope, the patient will feel the urge to defecate. This feeling may be relieved by having him breathe deeply but slowly with his mouth open. Dizziness or lightheadedness often occurs as a result of the head-down position and excessive deep breathing. The patient should be allowed to rest in a horizontal position for a few minutes before standing.

The position and the procedure may cause the patient to feel embarrassment and a loss of dignity. Assurance should be given that all efforts will be made to counteract this by adequate draping and the professional demeanor of the staff.

AFTERCARE

The physician should be contacted if rectal bleeding or severe abdominal pains occur.

PURPOSE Direct visualization of the large intestine through a fiberoptic colonoscope.

Because of the length of the colonoscope and its fiberoptic properties, a larger portion of the intestine can be directly visualized than is possible with proctosigmoidoscopy. Exclusive of surgery no other means exists by which this can be achieved. As colonoscopy has been available only since 1969, its practice is currently limited to large medical centers.

TIME The time required to perform colonoscopy is extremely variable. Although this can be accomplished within 30 minutes, it may require up to 3 hours if the tortuosity of the sigmoid colon and the angulation of the splenic and hepatic flexures make passage of the colonoscope difficult.

LOCATION Endoscopy suite or treatment room.

PERSONNEL Surgeon and assistant.

EQUIPMENT Colonoscope (Fig. 5-8). This instrument operates like other fiberoptic endoscopes (see pages 108–109).

PREPARATION 1. The patient's diet is limited to full fluids for 24 hours prior to the procedure. The evening before, a strong cathartic is taken, and at least 2 hours before the test, enemas are given.
2. Most patients are premedicated with sedatives or analgesics. Sufficient medication is given to relax the patient effectively without hindering his ability to cooperate with the examination.
3. When the examination is scheduled on an outpatient basis, the patient should be advised to come accompanied by

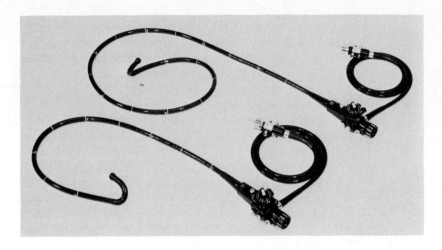

Figure 5-8. Fiberoptic colonoscope (shown in 105- and 185-cm lengths). (Courtesy Olympus Corporation of America, New Hyde Park, N.Y.)

someone who can assist him in returning home, especially if driving is necessary.

TECHNIQUE

1. Initial introduction of the colonoscope is accomplished with the patient in a left lateral recumbent position. It is often advantageous to change the patient's position to facilitate insertion into the transverse and ascending colon.
2. The colonoscope is passed its entire length. As it is slowly withdrawn, the intestinal mucosa is examined, suspect tissue removed for biopsy, specimens withdrawn for cytological study, and any polyps excised. Thus a definitive diagnosis may be made without resorting to a major abdominal operation.

PATIENT SENSATIONS

1. During the procedure air is insufflated to distend the lumen of the bowel and provide clearer visualization. This results in the patient's experiencing cramps. However, as the air is removed by the examiner or is rapidly expelled, this is only a transitory source of discomfort.
2. Although colonoscopy is not a particularly painful procedure, it is lengthy, tiring, and often difficult for the

patient to endure. This is further aggravated by embarrassment due to the nature of the procedure which requires close face-to-anus approximation and expulsion of insufflated air into the examiner's face.

AFTERCARE   1. The hospitalized patient will be returned to his room after completion of the examination. Vital signs should be checked and side rails raised until the medication has worn off.

2. If the procedure is done on an outpatient basis, the patient will be encouraged to rest until he feels able to leave.

Liver Biopsy

PURPOSE   To obtain a specimen of hepatic tissue for histological examination.

TIME   Ten minutes.

LOCATION   Patient's bedside.

PERSONNEL   Physician and assistant.

EQUIPMENT   Specialized biopsy needle and fixative agent.

TECHNIQUE
1. Liver biopsy may be done using an intercostal or a subcostal approach, the former being more common.
2. For the intercostal approach the patient lies in a supine position at the right edge of the bed. The right arm is raised and extended over the left shoulder behind the head, and the head is directed toward the left. This position provides maximal exposure of the right intercostal spaces (Fig. 5-9). For the subcostal approach the patient lies flat on his back.
3. The area chosen for biopsy is that of maximal hepatic dullness as determined by percussion. The skin is scrubbed with an antiseptic solution, draped with sterile

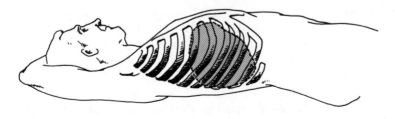

Figure 5-9. Patient position for intercostal approach to liver biopsy.

towels and infiltrated with a local anesthetic. The
anesthetic is then injected into the liver capsule.
4. Several types of needles are available for liver biopsy.
The two most commonly used are the Vim-Silverman
and the Menghini. The Menghini needle has the advantage
of being in the liver for less than 1 second as opposed to
the several seconds required with the Vim-Silverman
needle.
5. Before the biopsy needle enters the liver, the patient
is asked to hold his breath on expiration. He may resume
normal respiration immediately after the specimen of
liver tissue is withdrawn.

**PATIENT
SENSATIONS**
1. A stinging sensation will be experienced as the skin overlying the liver is infiltrated. Transitory pain is felt when
the anesthetic enters the liver capsule.
2. After the procedure the patient may have pain at the
puncture site, sometimes referred to the right shoulder,
but rarely lasting longer than 12 hours. Mild analgesics
are usually sufficient to control the pain.

PREPARATION
1. Before the procedure the patient must be evaluated to
ascertain that he is able to cooperate by holding his
breath when instructed.
2. Prothrombin time, bleeding time, and platelet count
are evaluated prior to the procedure. The biopsy is
contraindicated if any bleeding tendency or clotting
defect is present.
3. The patient's blood is typed and cross-matched; blood
is held on call.
4. The patient may be kept NPO.

AFTERCARE
1. Although uncommon, the most serious complication of
liver biopsy is hemorrhage. For this reason, the patient
lies on his right side for 1 hour after the procedure and
remains in bed for 24 hours.
2. He may be kept NPO until his condition has stabilized
and it is certain that no further medical or surgical intervention is necessary. Vital signs are assessed frequently
during the remainder of the day, and a hematocrit determination may be obtained if indicated.

Bibliography

Belinsky, I., Shinya, H., and Wolff, W. I. Colonofiberoscopy: Technique in colon examination. *Am. J. Nurs.* 73:306, 1973.

Beranbaum, S. L., and Meyers, P. H. *Special Procedures in Roentgen Diagnosis.* Springfield, Ill.: Thomas, 1964.

Beranbaum, S. L., and Yaghmai, M. *Fluoroscopy and Radiography of the Gastrointestinal Tract.* Wilmington, Del.: E. I. du Pont de Nemours and Co., 1967.

Berk, R. N. Radiology of the gallbladder and bile ducts. *Surg. Clin. North Am.* 53:973, 1973.

Bilbao, M. C., Frische, L. H., Dotter, C. T., and Rösch, J. Hypotonic duodenography. *Radiology* 89:438, 1967.

Eaton, S. B., Benedict, K. T., Jr., Ferucci, J. T., Jr., and Fleischli, D. J. Hypotonic duodenography. *Radiol. Clin. North Am.* 8:125, 1970.

Ferucci, J. T., Jr., and Eaton, S. B., Jr. Radiologic evaluation of obstructive jaundice. *Surg. Clin. North Am.* 54:573, 1974.

Fischer, M. G., Geffen, A., and Ozoktay, S. Z. Percutaneous transhepatic cholangiography. *Am. J. Gastroenterol.* 60:557, 1973.

Gregg, J. A., and Garabedian, M. Fiberoptic examination of the digestive tract. *Surg. Clin. North Am.* 51:633, 1971.

Gregg, J. A., and Garabedian, M. Esophageal endoscopy. *Surg. Clin. North Am.* 51:641, 1971.

Gregg, J. A., and Garabedian, M. Gastroscopy. *Surg. Clin. North Am.* 51:649, 1971.

Gregg, J. A., and Garabedian, M. Duodenoscopy. *Surg. Clin. North Am.* 51:657, 1971.

Loeb, P. M., Wheeler, H. O., and Berk, R. N. Endoscopic pancreatocholangiography in the diagnosis of biliary tract disease. *Surg. Clin. North Am.* 53:1007, 1973.

Margulis, A. R., and Burhenne, H. J. *Alimentary Tract Roentgenology* (2d ed.). St. Louis: Mosby, 1973.

Mujahed, Z., and Evans, J. A. Percutaneous transhepatic cholangiography. *Radiol. Clin. North Am.* 4:535, 1966.

Ogoshi, K., Niwa, M., Hara, Y., and Nebel, O. T. Endoscopic pancreatocholangiography in the evaluation of pancreatic and biliary disease. *Gastroenterology* 64:210, 1973.

Oi, I. Fiber duodenoscopy and endoscopic pancreatocholangiography. *Gastrointest. Endosc.* 17:59, 1970.

Sleisenger, M. H., and Fordham, J. S. *Gastrointestinal Disease.* Philadelphia: Saunders, 1973.

Spiro, H. M. *Clinical Gastroenterology.* New York: Macmillan, 1970.

Stauffer, M. Needle biopsy of the liver. *Surg. Clin. North Am.* 47:851, 1969.

Wolff, W. I., and Shinya, H. Colonofiberoscopy. *J.A.M.A.* 217:1509, 1971.

Wolff, W. I., Shinya, H., Geffen, A., and Ozaktay, S. Z. Colonofiberoscopy. *Am. J. Surg.* 123:180, 1972.

Cardiovascular System

6

Cardiac Catheterization

PURPOSE   Roentgenographic visualization of the chambers of the
heart and great vessels.

   The following can be accomplished with this examination:

1. Determination of intracardiac and intravascular pressures.
2. Determination of pulmonary blood flow and cardiac output.
3. Determination of oxygen content, saturation, and tension.
4. Detection of shunts.
5. Coronary artery visualization by injection of contrast material.
6. Visualization of the anatomy of cardiac chambers and identification of congenital anomalies and acquired valvular lesions.

TIME   Two to 3 hours depending on the information required.

LOCATION   Specialized cardiac catheterization laboratory where all the necessary equipment is readily available.

PERSONNEL   Cardiologist, radiologist, nurse, and technician. The physicians are gowned as for any sterile procedure.

EQUIPMENT   X-ray table (Fig. 6-1); fluoroscopy unit, cineradiograph, or rapid serial film changer; surgical instruments; radiopaque flexible catheters of various sizes; electrocardiograph; multi-channel recorder with oscilloscope for recording and reading pressure waves and the electrocardiogram; contrast material if angiocardiography is to be performed; and emergency equipment and medications for resuscitative measures.

   In place of an x-ray table a "cradle-top" table can be used which allows films to be taken in various degrees of obliquity by positioning the cradle rather than the patient. When this apparatus is used, the patient is secured with straps. With a routine x-ray table the patient is supported manually for oblique films.

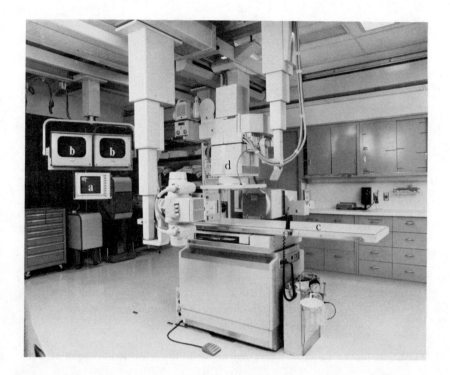

Figure 6-1. Cardiac catheterization laboratory. *a,* multichannel recorder; *b,* oscilloscope; *c,* x-ray table; *d,* fluoroscope. (Courtesy General Electric Company, Milwaukee, Wis.)

For the electrocardiogram, limb leads are placed on the patient before the procedure begins and the electrocardiogram is monitored throughout the examination.

TECHNIQUE

Cardiac catheterization may include a right heart study, left heart study, coronary arteriography, and angiocardiography. Although all four studies may be done at once, usually only those that pertain directly to the clinical problems are performed. In addition, cardiac output is routinely determined during cardiac catheterization.

A. Right heart catheterization

   1. The catheter is inserted into either an antecubital or a femoral vein.

2. It is passed through the inferior or superior vena cava (depending on its point of origin) and then advanced into the right atrium, right ventricle, pulmonary artery, and finally lodged in a small distal branch of the pulmonary artery (Fig. 6-2).

3. As the catheter traverses each of these areas, blood samples for oxygen analysis are taken and pressure recordings are made. Pressure gradients across the valves are routinely measured as this is the only way to determine the severity of a stenosis.

4. The various pressures measured throughout the procedure are transmitted through a transducer attached to the catheter. They appear as waves on the oscilloscope screen.

B. Left heart catheterization — this can be achieved by three methods:

1. Retrograde catheterization of the aorta
A second catheter is inserted through the femoral or brachial artery. The catheter is passed down the ascending aorta, across the aortic valve, and into the left ventricle (and sometimes into the left atrium) (Fig. 6-3). Again, pressure readings, pressure gradients, and blood samples are taken as the catheter passes through each area. The retrograde approach is the method of choice.

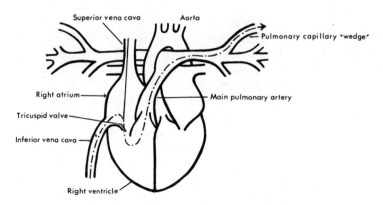

Figure 6-2. Catheter pathway for right heart catheterization *(dotted line).*

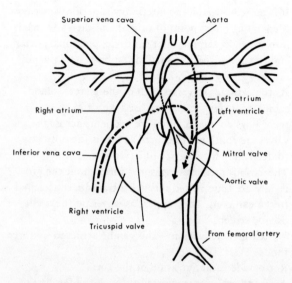

Figure 6-3. Catheter pathways for retrograde (*solid line*) and transseptal (*broken line*) approaches in left heart catheterization.

2. Transseptal puncture

   If stenosis of the aortic valve is present, it may be necessary to enter the left ventricle using a different approach. A catheter with a curved tip is inserted intravenously; the atrial septum is punctured and the catheter advanced to the left atrium and through the mitral valve into the left ventricle (see Fig. 6-3).

3. Direct puncture of the left ventricle may be necessary, although extremely rare.

C. Cardiac angiography

1. Coronary arteriography

   The arterial catheter is pulled back and relocated in one of the coronary arteries. When it is properly positioned, the contrast material is injected and recorded cineradiographically or by exposing multiple films in rapid sequence. The catheter is then repositioned in the second coronary artery. In this manner the vessels may be visualized, the collateral circulation demonstrated, and the degree of obstruction evaluated. Nitroglycerin may be administered prior to this portion of the procedure to prevent spasm and promote dilation of the coronary arteries.

2. Angiocardiography

Contrast material is injected into any of the four cardiac chambers to determine chamber size and the presence or absence of valvular stenosis or insufficiency and septal or valvular defects.

D. Cardiac output — this is measured by one of three methods:

1. Fick principle

The amount of blood flow through an organ (the lungs) is determined by substituting within an equation the total oxygen consumption and the difference in oxygen concentration of arterial and venous blood. To obtain these measurements, the patient's expired air is collected in a spirometer for 2 minutes. The volume and oxygen content are measured, and the oxygen consumption determined. Blood samples are withdrawn simultaneously from the pulmonary artery and a peripheral artery. These three determinants yield the pulmonary blood flow which equals the cardiac output (providing there are no shunts).

2. Indicator dilution method

A known amount of tracer dye, usually indocyanine green, is injected intravenously. Blood samples are drawn from a peripheral artery. The degree of dilution of the dye, which is a measure of blood flow, is perceived by a sensing device and recorded on the multi-channel oscilloscope as a curve; the curve corresponds to the cardiac output.

3. Thermodilution method

A known amount of iced solution such as dextrose in water is injected through the right heart catheter into the right atrium or superior vena cava. A temperature-sensing device in the catheter perceives the temperature change and the information is analyzed by a small computer which displays the cardiac output in digital form.

PATIENT
SENSATIONS

1. As various parts of the heart are stimulated by the catheter, extrasystoles may occur. This may be experienced by the patient as palpitations or a missed beat.

2. The contrast material used in angiography causes a sensation of warmth which varies in degree with the area injected. Other sensations, which occur and disappear rapidly, may also be experienced as a result of the contrast material. These symptoms may be categorized as follows:

   a. Pulmonary artery — searing heat, nausea, headache, and desire to cough.

   b. Coronary arteries — generalized warmth, nausea, headache, and chest pain.

   c. Aorta — nausea, headache, and an overwhelming surge of heat.

   d. Cardiac chambers — generalized warmth, nausea, and headache.

3. As the catheter is manipulated through a vessel, vasospasm may occur, causing severe pain.

4. Discomfort may result from lying flat for several hours, and anxiety may ensue from the continuous activity and cacophony surrounding the patient.

PREPARATION

1. Cardiac catheterization not only is an intrinsically difficult procedure for a patient to undergo but also is additionally demanding because of the implications of the findings. Therefore the patient facing the prospect of catheterization requires a great deal of explanation, reassurance, and understanding. A preliminary visit to the cardiac catheterization laboratory and meeting with the personnel involved with the procedure may help to assuage the patient's anxieties.

2. As the patient may experience nausea secondary to the contrast material, he remains fasting prior to the examination to prevent possible emesis and aspiration.

3. Dentures are removed.

4. The patient may receive sedation an hour before the procedure to control anxiety. Some physicians refrain from administering any medications because they may alter hemodynamics.

5. The patient should report to the cardiologist any pain or discomfort experienced during the procedure.

AFTERCARE

1. Vital signs are monitored frequently after the patient returns to his unit until his condition has stabilized.
2. Pulses should be taken apically. Although arrhythmias more commonly occur during the procedure, they may become evident after its completion. Arrhythmias are more easily discernible apically.
3. Bed rest is maintained for 12 hours following the procedure.
4. The arterial puncture site should be checked for bleeding and swelling. These signs may indicate acute hematoma formation. If they occur, firm pressure cephalad to the puncture site should be applied and medical assistance summoned.
5. Pulses distal to the punctured arterial vessel should be checked frequently. Sudden pain associated with cold, white, blotchy skin is indicative of vascular insufficiency probably secondary to embolization and requires immediate intervention.
6. A complication of the venous approach (as in a right heart study) is thrombophlebitis in the involved extremity. The area should be checked for warmth, pain, swelling, and redness, and appropriate therapeutic measures instituted.

Peripheral, Thoracic, and Abdominal Angiography

PURPOSE

Visualization of peripheral or visceral vessels to:
1. Evaluate abnormalities of vascular structure and function.
2. Identify mass lesions by observation of vessel displacement and abnormal areas of vascularity.
3. Identify bleeding sites and infuse drugs selectively.

All four extremities and the major organs supplied by the thoracic and abdominal aorta may be studied with this technique. Common studies are of the lower extremities; the kidneys, pancreas, and spleen; the portal system; and the GI tract (Fig. 6-4).

TIME

Thirty minutes to 3 hours. Variables determining time include the age of the patient, the status of the vasculature, and the problem under investigation.

LOCATION

Radiology department.

PERSONNEL

Radiologist and assistants gowned as for any sterile procedure.

EQUIPMENT

X-ray table, fluoroscopy unit, rapid-sequence film changer or cineradiograph, radiopaque catheters.

TECHNIQUE

1. The patient is placed in a supine position on the x-ray table. Restraints may be applied if the patient is unable to cooperate and there is difficulty in maintaining the sterile field or the position of the needle or catheter. An intravenous infusion may be started at this time to provide an easily accessible route for medication and to maintain hydration during the procedure.
2. Regardless of the organ to be studied, the femoral artery is usually the preferred point of entry. However, if these arteries are tortuous, atherosclerotic, or congenitally defective in some way, the axillary artery may be chosen as the puncture site.

134

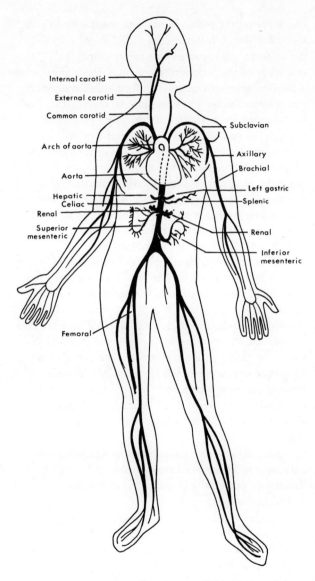

Figure 6-4. Diagram of major arteries studied during angiography.

3. The skin over the puncture site is cleansed with an anti-septic solution, infiltrated with a local anesthetic, and the adjacent areas covered with sterile drapes.

4. In a study of the peripheral circulation, the femoral artery is usually punctured and the contrast material injected through the needle. For other arterial studies, the needle is exchanged for a catheter by inserting a guide wire through the needle and passing the catheter over the guide wire. Under fluoroscopic guidance the catheter is advanced to the vessel to be studied.

5. When the needle or catheter is accurately positioned, it is taped in place and attached to an automatic injector. The injector is a machine which can be set to deliver a certain amount of contrast material in a specific period of time, as determined by the radiologist.

6. The contrast material is automatically injected and rapid-sequence films are taken. The films will usually demonstrate all phases of circulation — arterial, capillary, and venous.

7. If the organ under investigation is supplied by more than one branch of the aorta, for example, the pancreas, it will be necessary either to reposition the catheter and repeat the injection and filming or initially to insert femoral catheters bilaterally.

8. If special views are required to clarify visualization, either the patient or the x-ray equipment may be re-positioned.

9. Pharmacoangiography and superselective angiography are recent refinements of angiographic technique. Both will clearly extend the length of the procedure.
   a. Pharmacoangiography
      By injecting vasodilators or vasoconstrictors, or both, in combination with the contrast medium, the arterial blood flow — and thus the flow of contrast material — is manipulated in such a way as to supply greater detail of the organ under study.
   b. Superselective angiography
      The catheter is advanced beyond the major supplying artery into its branches to obtain even more specific information about the nature of the problem.

10. Throughout the examination, the patient is observed for alterations in cardiovascular status. This may be accomplished by frequent blood pressure readings, electrocardiographic monitoring, and checking of peripheral pulses.

11. At the conclusion of the procedure, the needle or catheter is removed and firm, steady pressure is applied to the puncture site. Before the patient is returned to his room the site is carefully observed to ensure that there is no hematoma formation. A pressure dressing is usually applied.

PATIENT SENSATIONS

The patient may experience:

1. A stinging sensation from injection of the local anesthetic agent.

2. Discomfort from maintaining one position for an extended period of time.

3. Discomfort and frustration if restraints have been applied.

4. A transient feeling of extreme heat on injection of the contrast material in the distribution of the vessel being injected.

5. Pain, depending on the exact vessel under study. The radiologist will forewarn the patient of the precise nature and severity of the pain.

6. Embarrassment from preprocedure shaving of the groin and from the brief exposure of the groin area prior to placement of the drapes.

7. Postprocedure discomfort at the puncture site.

PREPARATION

1. The hematological status of the patient is evaluated. Anticoagulant therapy may be discontinued the day before the procedure and vitamin K or protamine sulfate administered. The anemic patient may be transfused.

2. When a femoral or axillary approach is planned, both groins or the left or right axilla is usually shaved and cleansed with an antiseptic solution.

3. If the area to be visualized may be obscured by the presence of gas or feces in the bowel, diet may be altered and cathartics may be administered. The exact protocol varies with the institution.

4. Present thinking tends toward maintenance of oral hydration before and during the procedure unless surgery is anticipated to follow immediately.
5. All metallic objects which might lie within the field of visualization should be removed. These include such items as watches, rings, necklaces, and religious objects. Metal is radiopaque and will interfere with accurate interpretation of the films.
6. A baseline record of vital signs should be obtained before the patient is premedicated to provide a means of post-procedure comparison.
7. The appropriate peripheral pulses should be located and the skin marked beforehand to provide ease in locating and evaluating them after the procedure.
8. Premedication usually consists of a combination of a sedative and an analgesic. The objective is to relax the patient without interfering with his ability to cooperate during the procedure.
9. The patient should report to the radiologist any pain or discomfort experienced during the procedure.
10. Since radiopaque contrast material is an osmotic diuretic, it is desirable to have the patient void just before being sent for the study. This minimizes discomfort due to an overdistended bladder during the procedure.

AFTERCARE

1. Vital signs should be monitored at frequent intervals until they stabilize at or near the baseline values. If an axillary artery was the puncture site, blood pressures should be measured contralaterally to prevent obliteration of the pulses distal to the site.
2. Application of cold to the puncture site decreases the possibility of hematoma formation.
3. The puncture site should be checked for swelling and bleeding, which may be indicative of hematoma formation. If this becomes evident, pressure cephalad to the puncture site should be applied and medical assistance summoned.
4. Evaluation of the adequacy of peripheral circulation is crucial. A hematoma or embolization to a distal artery may diminish or occlude circulation to an extremity.

The presence of peripheral pulses should be ascertained frequently and compared with the baseline. The color and temperature of the involved extremity should be noted.

5. Bed rest is maintained for 12 to 24 hours following the procedure.

Lower Extremity Phlebography
(Venography)

PURPOSE   Roentgenographic visualization of the venous system of the
lower extremities.

This procedure is performed primarily to determine
venous competence and the presence and degree of thrombosis. Although phlebography may be performed to evaluate
venous circulation of the upper extremities and visceral
organs, it is used most frequently to examine the lower
extremities and only that study will be discussed here.

TIME   Five to 30 minutes depending on the technique utilized.

LOCATION   Radiology department.

PERSONNEL   Radiologist and technician.

EQUIPMENT   Tilting x-ray table, fluoroscopy unit, and overhead radiographic apparatus.

PREPARATION None.

TECHNIQUE   1. The choice of injection site is determined by the information sought and the ease with which it can be obtained.
   a. Percutaneous ascending venography involves the intro-
      duction of contrast material into a vein on the dorsal
      surface of the foot. It is the most common approach.
   b. Percutaneous femoral venography involves the injection
      of contrast material into the venous system via the
      femoral vein. It is often done to achieve more satis-
      factory opacification of the external and common iliac
      veins and the inferior vena cava than is possible with
      percutaneous ascending venography.
2. The patient's position will range from supine to various
   degrees of elevation from the horizontal depending on
   the technique used.

3. Tourniquets may be placed above the ankle or the knee and sometimes on the contralateral thigh to control filling and improve deep-vein opacification. Extensive varices may be compressed by an Ace bandage.

4. Although a cutdown may sometimes be necessary, venipuncture is usually accomplished with a scalp vein needle.

5. The extremities may be studied singly, consecutively, or simultaneously.

6. When the femoral approach is used, the skin and subcutaneous tissues are first infiltrated with a local anesthetic.

7. Contrast material is either manually injected or instilled by infusion. Opacification is observed fluoroscopically and appropriate spot films are taken. At or just before the completion of the injection, any tourniquets in use are removed.

8. Overhead radiographs are then obtained. During this period the patient may be asked to perform various activities such as pushing down with his foot against the examiner's hand, lying prone with his leg flexed, or executing a Valsalva maneuver. These are all measures to improve the rate and completeness of venous filling.

9. On completion of filming, the patient is returned to the horizontal position. The contrast medium is removed from the venous system either by injection of normal saline or by exercise, elevation, or massage of the extremity. Removal of the contrast agent is necessary because its irritating effect on the intima of the veins may cause phlebitis.

10. The needle or needles are removed and pressure is applied. If a cutdown was necessary, the site is sutured and a sterile dressing applied.

PATIENT SENSATIONS

1. Insertion of the needle in the foot or groin will cause a sensation similar to that of venipuncture.

2. Local anesthetic infiltration will cause first the sensation of venipuncture, then a mild, transitory burning sensation, and finally a feeling of numbness.

3. During injection of the contrast material the patient will feel a localized burning pain persisting for 2 to 3 minutes

due to the irritating effect of the contrast material and its distension of the vessels. This is usually followed by a transient sensation of warmth throughout the body when the contrast medium becomes disseminated in the systemic circulation.

4. Some degree of flushing, headache, nausea, or vomiting, or any combination of these, is commonly experienced.

5. A small percentage of patients may have a syncopal attack as a result of the vasodilatory effect of the contrast material, the semiupright position necessary for the study, and the degree of venous incompetence present. Any warning of such an attack should be reported to the physician.

6. The use of tourniquets may cause the patient pain.

AFTERCARE

1. Periods of elevation of the extremity should alternate with frequent periods of walking to remove all contrast material, which might pool in varicosities.

2. Extravasation of contrast material from a ruptured vein may occur, causing swelling. Treatment includes elevation of the extremity and application of heat. The latter will increase circulation to the area and hasten absorption of the extravasated contrast material.

3. The temperature and color of the extremities should be evaluated regularly. Coolness and pale or dusky color are signs of venous occlusion.

4. Sterile dressing technique should be carried out at the cutdown site to prevent the development of a local infection.

Bibliography

Abrams, H. R. (Ed.). *Angiography* (2d ed.). Boston: Little, Brown, 1971.

Ekelund, L., and Lunderquist, A. Pharmacoangiography with angiotensin. *Radiology* 110:533, 1974.

Friedberg, C. K. *Diseases of the Heart* (3d ed.). Philadelphia: Saunders, 1966.

Hurst, J. W. (Ed.). *The Heart, Arteries, and Veins* (3d ed.). New York: McGraw-Hill, 1974.

Kernicki, J., Bullock, B., and Matthews, J. *Cardiovascular Nursing.* New York: Putnam, 1970.

Lamberton, M. M. Cardiac catheterization: Anticipatory nursing care. *Am. J. Nurs.* 71:1718, 1971.

Lea, T. M. Phlebography. *Arch. Surg.* 104:145, 1972.

Luisada, A. A. (Ed.). *Examination of the Cardiac Patient.* New York: McGraw-Hill, 1965.

O'Connell, N. D. Venography. *Radiography* 39:211, 1973.

Rabinov, K., and Paulin, S. Roentgen diagnosis of venous thrombosis in the leg. *Arch. Surg.* 104:134, 1972.

Schobinger, R. A., and Ruzicka, F. F. *Vascular Roentgenology.* New York: Macmillan, 1964.

Wise, R. E., and Johnston, D. O. The role of angiography in the evaluation of surgical patients. *Surg. Clin. North Am.* 50:645, 1970.

7

Respiratory System

Bronchoscopy

PURPOSE Direct visualization of the tracheobronchial tree for diagnostic or therapeutic purposes.
1. Diagnostic
   a. Tissue biopsy, e.g., tumor or diseased membrane.
   b. Aspiration of secretions for smear and culture studies, e.g., bacteriological, fungal, cytological.
   c. Identification of site of hemorrhage in unexplained hemoptysis.
   d. Determination of degree and cause of tracheal stenosis in cases of upper airway obstruction.
2. Therapeutic
   a. Removal of foreign body or localized lesion.
   b. Aspiration of obstructing secretions (to relieve atelectasis).
   c. Drainage of abscesses.

TIME Fifteen to 30 minutes. An additional 15 minutes are usually required to achieve adequate anesthesia.

PERSONNEL Physician (endoscopist), assistant to position the head, scrub nurse, circulating nurse, and anesthesiologist (if general anesthesia is used). The endoscopist and scrub nurse wear sterile gown and gloves, cap, and mask. All others wear only a cap and mask.

LOCATION Endoscopy suite, operating room, intensive care unit, or emergency room.

ROOM AND EQUIPMENT Endoscopy suite, bronchoscope, forceps, lighted telescope, and fiberoptic bronchoscope.
   The endoscopy suite is essentially an operating room, with all the associated equipment, including the means to administer anesthesia, oxygen, and suction, and an emergency cart.

The standard bronchoscope is a hollow metal tube with a distal light and a tube incorporated in the wall of the bronchoscope for administration of oxygen or anesthetic gases, if necessary (Fig. 7-1). It is available in various diameters and lengths. The patient breathes through and around the scope; therefore the airway is in no way compromised.

Forceps of various shapes and designs are used for biopsies and removal of foreign bodies. Lighted telescopes may be passed through a bronchoscope, thus permitting visualization of areas at angles other than the forward view.

Fiberoptic bronchoscopes allow the endoscopist to view and remove specimens in the bronchial segments not accessible to the usually straight, rigid scopes. Fiberoptic bronchoscopes are fully flexible, providing an undistorted image even when completely bent. The image is transmitted through a series of fiberglass bundles. Illumination is provided by an external light source and conducted through a second set of fiber bundles. By rotation of the scope and flexion of the tip, the bronchoscope may be introduced into all segments

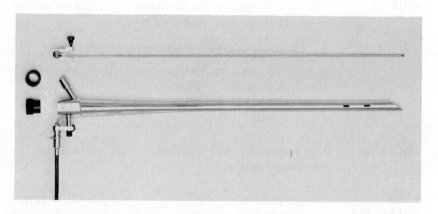

Figure 7-1. The standard rigid bronchoscope consists of a hollow metal tube with a distal light and an integral tube for administering oxygen or anesthetic gases. (Courtesy American Cystoscope Makers, Inc., Stamford, Conn.)

of the tracheobronchial tree. Because of the flexible
nature of this instrument, patients can be examined in
virtually any position and need not assume the posture
necessary for an examination with the rigid bronchoscope.
This provides greater ease for both the patient and the
examiner (Fig. 7-2).

Fiberoptic bronchoscopes are much narrower than the
rigid bronchoscopes and therefore can be passed through
the endotracheal tube of patients on mechanical ventilators.
Their flexibility offers direct visualization of upper lobe
segments and permits brush biopsy of all segments under
direct vision. They offer the further advantage of examination of a patient, under local anesthesia, at the bedside. However, since biopsy forceps must be passed through a small
aspiration channel, the size of the biopsy specimen is smaller
than that obtained with the rigid bronchoscope. Furthermore,
foreign body removal or resection of localized lesions is often
not possible.

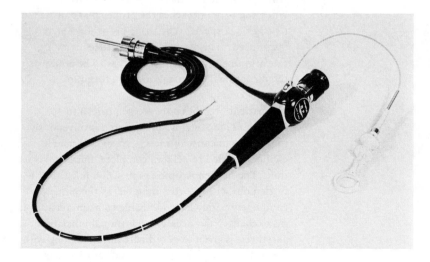

Figure 7-2. The fiberoptic bronchoscope is flexible and permits visualization
of areas inaccessible to the rigid bronchoscope. (Courtesy Olympus Corporation of America, New Hyde Park, N. Y.)

TECHNIQUE   **A.** Anesthesia

Either topical or general anesthesia may be used. Although topical anesthesia is preferable, general anesthesia is necessary for very apprehensive patients or those in whom a topical anesthetic is not effective.

1. Topical anesthesia

    Lidocaine or a similar agent is administered by spraying the mouth, pharynx, and hypopharynx. Additional anesthetic is dropped by syringe and cannula onto the larynx and then through the larynx to the tracheobronchial tree. The same effect may be achieved by other methods such as gargling. Approximately 10 to 15 minutes are required to obtain adequate anesthesia.

2. General anesthesia

    All patients receiving a general anesthetic will have an intravenous infusion and most will have electrocardiographic monitoring. Anesthesia may be induced by either of two methods.

    a. Inhalation technique

        Any one of the anesthetic gases may be used. When the patient reaches the proper plane of relaxation, a special ventilating bronchoscope is introduced. This bronchoscope is fitted with a side arm to allow the anesthetic gas to be administered continually throughout the procedure.

    b. Apneic technique

        The patient breathes pure oxygen for 10 to 15 minutes. Thiopental is administered intravenously to produce unconsciousness; curare or succinylcholine is added to achieve complete muscle relaxation. The bronchoscopic examination must then be carried out within 2 to 3 minutes, as the patient is completely paralyzed and unable to maintain adequate gas exchange. On occasion, additional inhalation anesthetic is given to coordinate his awakening with the restoration of muscle tone and spontaneous respiration.

B. Position

The patient is placed in a dorsal recumbent position with his head extended over the end of the table. An assistant positions and supports the head so that it is slightly extended and elevated. When the bronchoscope passes into the trachea, the head may be lowered slightly and moved from side to side to permit passage of the endoscope sequentially into the two main bronchi. When a fiberoptic bronchoscope is used this position is not necessary — the patient may be lying or sitting.

C. Examination

The bronchoscopic examination includes observation of the position of the trachea, the status of the mucosal lining, and the character of secretions. The carina is checked for position and mobility. A systematic review is done of the major and secondary bronchi noting the color, the mucosal changes and the presence or absence of lesions. Suspect tissue is removed for study and secretions aspirated for laboratory analysis. Washings may also be obtained by instillation and subsequent aspiration of small aliquots of normal saline solution.

PATIENT SENSATIONS

1. Local anesthesia

The application of the local anesthetic is often the most difficult part of the procedure for the patient. The gag and cough reflexes are stimulated, causing associated discomforts. Also, the patient will feel as if his tongue and throat are swollen. Although swallowing is unimpaired, the patient will feel as if he is unable to swallow. Suctioning is done intermittently throughout the procedure to aspirate the collected secretions. The patient will note pressure of the bronchoscope at the major points of contact with the scope — the side of the mouth, the throat, and the larynx. Discomfort is minimal if he is confident that the airway will not be blocked. Confidence will contribute to relaxation, which is essential for completion of the examination.

2. General anesthesia

The patient will experience no sensation while under general anesthesia. However, pressure points may be felt after the anesthetic wears off, but to a lesser degree than when local anesthesia is used. The patient will have the usual aftereffects of general anesthesia. If succinylcholine or curare is used, myalgias may be felt the following day.

PREPARATION

1. The patient should be reassured that the airway will in no way be obstructed.
2. A fasting state is maintained to prevent aspiration during the procedure.
3. Dentures and jewelry are removed.
4. Nail polish is removed if the procedure is carried out under general anesthesia.
5. Premedication usually includes a combination of barbiturates, narcotic analgesics, and tranquilizers to control anxiety and ensure relaxation during the procedure. Atropine may also be administered to control copious secretions and prevent reflex bradycardia.

AFTERCARE

1. Vital signs are monitored until they are stable.
2. When the procedure is done under local anesthesia, the patient may not eat or drink until the cough and gag reflexes have returned. This usually requires 1 1/2 hours.
3. After general anesthesia, oral intake is permitted only when the patient has regained full consciousness and bowel sounds are present.
4. After a biopsy, some hemoptysis is expected.
5. The patient should be observed for the following complications:
   a. Hemorrhage.
   b. Respiratory distress, e.g., wheezing, dyspnea, cyanosis, tachypnea, hypertension, tachycardia, or stridor.
   c. Elevated temperature.
6. Sputum should be collected for the 24 hours immediately following bronchoscopy for cytological studies and culture.

Laryngoscopy

PURPOSE   Direct visualization of the larynx for diagnostic or therapeutic purposes.
1. Diagnostic
   a. Removal of tissue for biopsy.
   b. Evaluation of laryngeal function, e.g., vocal cord
      paralysis.
   c. Determination of the presence or absence of inflamma-
      tion.
2. Therapeutic
   a. Removal of lesions, e.g., polyps or granulomas.
   b. Removal of foreign bodies.
   c. Dilation of laryngeal strictures.
   d. Application of therapeutic modalities, e.g., laser beams.

TIME
PERSONNEL } Refer to the section on bronchoscopy (page 147).
LOCATION

EQUIPMENT Laryngoscope. The standard laryngoscope is a hollow metal
tube with a distal light source (Fig. 7-3). It is available in
various diameters and lengths.

TECHNIQUE As in bronchoscopy either local or general anesthesia is used.
Local anesthesia is generally preferred. Vocal cord motility
can be viewed only when the patient is awake and able to
phonate. When the patient is particularly anxious or has
a strong gag reflex, general anesthesia is employed.
    Refer to bronchoscopy procedure for details concerning
anesthesia induction and patient position.

PATIENT   Refer to bronchoscopy procedure.
SENSATIONS

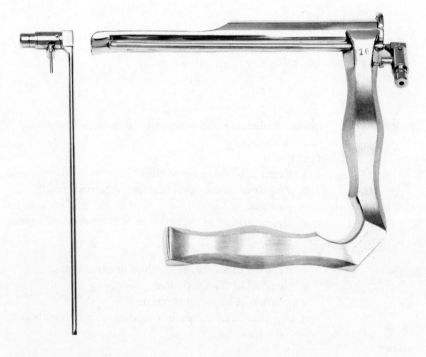

Figure 7-3. Jackson laryngoscope. (Courtesy American Cystoscope Makers, Inc., Stamford, Conn.)

PREPARATION Refer to bronchoscopy procedure. The only difference is the addition of a belladonna derivative (e.g., atropine) to reduce secretions.

AFTERCARE Refer to bronchoscopy procedure. In addition, the patient should be observed for respiratory stridor secondary to edema.

Bronchography

PURPOSE Roentgenographic visualization of the bronchial tree.
This procedure is usually performed to delineate the extent of known disease, such as bronchiectasis, or to localize and document suspected disease.

TIME One hour. The examination may be longer if satisfactory anesthesia is difficult to achieve or the patient has difficulty tolerating the procedure.

LOCATION Radiology department.

PERSONNEL Radiologist and technician.

EQUIPMENT Fluoroscopy unit, overhead x-ray apparatus, and tilting x-ray table.

TECHNIQUE Topical anesthesia is used. Variations exist from one hospital to another in methods of induction. Generally, the pharynx, hypopharynx, tonsil area, and epiglottis are sprayed and swabbed with the anesthetic solution. After a short wait, additional amounts of the anesthetic agent are dropped through the glottis by means of a cannula and syringe. This stimulates coughing, which distributes the anesthetic. Other methods of administering the anesthetic include intermittent positive pressure breathing and use of an ultrasonic nebulizer.
Once satisfactory anesthesia has been achieved, a soft, pliable catheter is inserted via the nose or mouth through the larynx to the bifurcation of the trachea. This is carried out under fluoroscopic control with the patient in an upright or semiupright position on the x-ray table. This method is called *transglottic catheterization,* and although other methods are in use, it is the most common.

The catheter is advanced into the bronchus on the side to be studied. Contrast material is injected through the catheter during the expiratory phase of respiration. The patient is instructed to inhale deeply to spread the contrast material uniformly throughout the lung. By rotating the patient into various positions and tilting the table, the entire bronchial tree can be visualized. Spot films are taken depending on what is seen fluoroscopically.

After the fluoroscopic examination is completed, several overhead radiographs are exposed. The patient is returned to the sitting position and encouraged to cough vigorously in order to expectorate the contrast material. Posttussive films are then obtained.

If both lungs must be examined, the physician may elect to study the second side at a later date.

PREPARATION
1. Oral intake is prohibited for several hours before the procedure to prevent aspiration during the examination.
2. Premedication is administered 30 to 45 minutes before procedure to allay anxiety, suppress coughing, and control secretions. An example of a premedication combination is meperidine, codeine sulfate, and atropine sulfate.
3. If secretions are copious, postural drainage may need to be performed for up to several days before the test, as excessive bronchial secretions may interfere with anesthesia induction and contrast filling.

PATIENT SENSATIONS
1. Even with maximal cooperation on the part of the patient, this procedure is traumatic and physically and emotionally taxing. It might be beneficial for a staff member with whom the patient is familiar and comfortable to accompany him to offer support and encouragement.
2. Until the catheter has passed through the larynx, the gag and cough reflexes are stimulated. The patient may retch and cough vigorously throughout this portion of the procedure. As a result of the local anesthetic, the patient may feel as if his tongue and throat are swollen.
3. Once the catheter has passed the larynx, there is less discomfort until it reaches more distal structures, when there is a tendency to cough. Panting will help suppress

the cough. This should be emphasized, as coughing may displace the catheter and prevent adequate examination.

AFTERCARE
1. Oral intake is not permitted until the cough and gag reflexes have returned.
2. Coughing is encouraged to rid the bronchial tree of the contrast material. Chest physical therapy may also be necessary.
3. The patient's temperature should be monitored regularly for 24 hours, as the contrast material may block the very distal bronchioles and cause atelectasis or pneumonitis.

Thoracentesis

PURPOSE
Removal of fluid from the pleural cavity for diagnostic or therapeutic purposes.

1. Diagnostic — to obtain specimens for:
   a. Bacteriological study (e.g., smears and cultures for bacteria and fungi).
   b. Complete and differential cell counts.
   c. Gross appearance (e.g., bloody, purulent, serous, or chylous).
   d. Specific gravity.
   e. Cytological study.
   f. Smears and cultures for acid-fast bacilli.
   g. Biochemical analysis (e.g., glucose, lactic dehydrogenase, amylase, and protein).
   h. In some instances: LE cell preparation, rheumatoid arthritis factor, antinuclear antibody, viral titers.

   When thoracentesis is performed for diagnostic purposes, approximately 20 ml of fluid is removed.

2. Therapeutic — to relieve respiratory distress. The amount of fluid removed at any one time is usually limited to 1 to 2 liters. If additional fluid is present, another puncture is performed at a later time.

TIME
Ten minutes. If it is necessary to remove a large amount of fluid, the length of the procedure will necessarily be extended.

LOCATION
Treatment room or patient's bedside.

PERSONNEL
Physician and assistant.

EQUIPMENT
Specialized needle, three-way stopcock, appropriate specimen containers, and large sterile receptacle.

158

TECHNIQUE   The patient sits with his feet dangling over the side of the bed or the examining table. A pillow is placed on the bedside table on which the patient rests his arms and head; the arms are crossed to afford maximal exposure of the intercostal spaces.

The puncture site is chosen by x-ray study and by percussion of the chest to determine the area of maximal dullness. The skin is swabbed with an antiseptic solution, sterile drapes are placed on adjacent areas, and an anesthetic solution is injected. Once the area has been adequately anesthetized, the needle is inserted into the predetermined interthoracic space. If the procedure is being performed for diagnostic purposes, a 20-ml syringe is attached to the needle and the necessary fluid is aspirated. If it is necessary to withdraw a large volume of fluid, a three-way stopcock is affixed to the needle. Attached to the remaining two outlets are a 50-ml syringe and a length of sterile tubing which is joined to a collecting bottle.

After the necessary fluid has been removed, the needle is withdrawn and a Band-Aid applied over the puncture site.

PREPARATION   As excessive coughing may cause displacement of the needle or perforation of the pleura, an antitussive medication may be administered. The patient should also be instructed to pant slowly in order to suppress coughing.

PATIENT SENSATIONS

1. As the anesthetic solution is being injected, the patient will experience a mild burning sensation.
2. As the parietal pleura is infiltrated, a sharp transitory pain may be felt.
3. If adequate anesthesia has been employed, the patient will feel only the pressure of the needle as it is inserted but no pain.
4. A pulling sensation or a desire to cough may be experienced as the needle is removed at the end of the procedure. These sensations are related to reexpansion of the lung.
5. If a large volume of fluid is withdrawn, the patient should realize considerable respiratory relief.

AFTERCARE   A follow-up chest x-ray is obtained to ascertain that a pneu-
mothorax has not occurred as a result of inadvertent introduction of air or puncture of the lung. The patient should
be observed for changes in respiration, pulse, and color.
Coughing or the appearance of blood-tinged sputum should
also be noted.

Pulmonary Function Tests (PFTs)

PURPOSE Detecting of abnormalities in pulmonary function.

These tests are an adjunct to other clinical studies. The objective measurements provided by these tests indicate the presence and nature of an abnormality, i.e., obstructive versus restrictive disease and the degree of severity. The results are not pathognomonic of any specific lesion.

The primary uses of the tests are to evaluate pulmonary status preoperatively, particularly in patients undergoing thoracic surgery, and to follow the course of a pulmonary disease and determine the efficacy of treatment.

TIME Extremely variable. The duration of the procedure depends on the number of measurements carried out. Extensive testing may require up to 2 hours but is not routinely performed.

LOCATION Pulmonary function laboratory, physician's office, or patient's bedside.

PERSONNEL Technician, nurse, or physician.

EQUIPMENT The basic equipment used is a spirometer. The patient breathes into an attached mouthpiece. Normally spirometers have bellows which are displaced by the patient's respiratory effort or consist of a drum inverted over water. As the patient inhales, the volume of gas in the drum decreases; as he exhales, the volume of gas in the drum increases. A pen and paper (kymograph) are attached to the spirometer and record the motions graphically. During most of the testing, the patient wears nose clips. This ensures mouth breathing and prevents air leakage. Figure 7-4 shows this equipment in use.

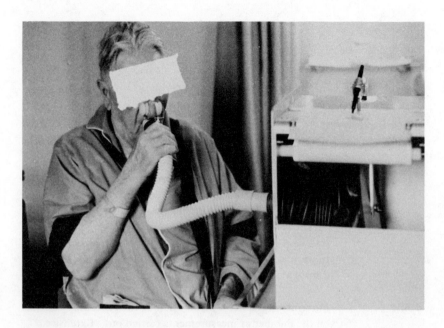

Figure 7-4. Setup for pulmonary function testing showing patient with nose clips and mouthpiece in position, side of spirometer open to expose bellows and kymograph atop spirometer.

TECHNIQUE   Both lung volumes and flow rates may be assessed.

A. Lung volumes

There are four volumes and four capacities, the latter consisting of two or more volumes.

Tidal volume (TV) — amount of air inhaled or exhaled during one respiratory cycle.

Inspiratory reserve volume (IRV) — maximal amount of air that can be inspired from the end inspiratory level (after a normal inspiration).

Expiratory reserve volume (ERV) — maximal amount of air that can be expired from the end expiratory level (after a normal expiration).

Residual volume (RV) — volume of air remaining in the lungs after maximal expiration.

Vital capacity (VC) — volume of air that can be force-
fully exhaled following a maximal inspiration or
inhaled following a maximal expiration (VC = TV +
IRV + ERV).

Inspiratory capacity (IC) — maximal amount of air
that can be inspired from an end expiration (IC =
TV + IRV).

Total lung capacity (TLC) — volume of air in the lungs
following a maximal inspiration (TLC = TV + IRV +
ERV + RV).

Functional residual capacity (FRC) — volume of air
remaining in the lungs from the end expiratory level
(FRC = ERV + RV).

After the patient is seated next to the spirometer, nose
clips are applied and he is asked to place his lips tightly
around the mouthpiece. He is instructed to breathe normally
(TV). After a normal inspiration, he is asked to keep breathing in until his lungs are completely filled (IRV). After a
normal expiration, he is asked to force out all of the air in
his lungs (ERV). From these three determinations, vital
capacity and inspiratory capacity can be calculated.

Residual volume, functional residual capacity, and total
lung capacity cannot be measured by direct spirometry. The
indirect methods for determining these values include the
closed circuit method, the open circuit method, and plethysmography.

1. Closed circuit method
   A known amount of an insoluble gas such as helium is
   mixed with air and put in the spirometer. The patient
   rebreathes the mixture until the concentration of helium
   is equal in both the lungs and the spirometer. A meter
   records the concentration within the spirometer. From
   a series of equations the initial volume of gas in the lungs
   can then be calculated.

2. Open circuit method
   The nitrogen washout technique is an example of the
   open circuit method. The patient breathes 100% oxygen
   for several minutes, thus washing out the nitrogen from
   the lungs. The expired gas is collected and measured for

its volume and nitrogen concentration. Since alveolar air is known to contain 80% nitrogen, the total amount of air in the lungs can be computed. Healthy adults usually wash out all the nitrogen within 2 to 3 minutes. Patients with obstructive disease require a longer period.

3. Plethysmography

The plethysmograph ("body box") is about the size of a telephone booth. It has sufficient room for the patient to sit. The portion over the patient's head is transparent so that he can always be seen by the examiner. With the box closed, there is an airtight system. The volume of gas in the body box is known. As volume and pressure vary inversely, the volumes of gas in the lung can be computed by measuring the pressure changes produced as the patient breathes in the body box.

B. Flow rates

1. Forced expiratory volume (FEV) — volume of air that can be expired in 1, 2, or 3 seconds (FEV_1, FEV_2, FEV_3). FEV_1 is one of the most important determinants in evaluating the mechanics of expiration.

2. Maximum expiratory flow rate (MEFR) and maximum midexpiratory flow rate (MMFR) are determined from the FEV and expressed in liters per minute.

The patient is asked to inspire maximally and then then exhale as fast, hard, and long as he can. Thus the FEV_1, FEV_2, and FEV_3 are determined. This maneuver is repeated several times and the best value taken. By utilizing different parts of the slope produced graphically from the FEV, the MEFR and MMFR can also be determined. When these values demonstrate obstruction, this test may be repeated after the administration of bronchodilators. This will usually demonstrate whether or not the obstruction is reversible. In some patients, however, reversibility can be demonstrated only after several days of oral or parenteral bronchodilators.

3. Maximum inspiratory flow rate (MIFR) — speed at which a maximal inspiration is taken, reported in liters per minute. To calculate the MIFR, the patient is asked to breathe in as deeply and rapidly as he can.

4. Maximum voluntary ventilation (MVV) — maximal amount of air that can be breathed in 1 minute. The MVV is determined by having the patient breathe as deeply and rapidly as he can for 15 seconds through a mouthpiece attached to a three-way valve; to the valve is connected a Douglas bag so that all expired air is collected. Multiplying the volume of air collected by 4 gives the MVV in liters per minute.

Arterial blood gas values may be obtained with the patient at rest and after exercise. The spirometric tests may also be done during exercise. Methods of exercise during the tests include stepping up and down a raised platform for several minutes or using a bicycle ergometer which permits pre-setting of the level of work to be expended.

PATIENT SENSATIONS

1. When complete testing is done in the pulmonary function laboratory, the array of complex equipment may increase the patient's anxiety.
2. If extensive testing is done, the patient will be fatigued from the necessity of continued concentration and exertion of effort.
3. If the body plethysmograph is used, the patient may feel claustrophobic and uncomfortably warm.
4. Patients, particularly those with compromised pulmonary function, often complain of a feeling of suffocation with the nose clips in place.
5. Arterial puncture is painful.

PREPARATION

1. Success and accuracy of some pulmonary function tests depend on the effort exerted by the patient. Therefore his understanding and cooperation are crucial.
2. Loose clothing should be worn during the testing. Any garment that restricts thoracic expansion such as a belt or girdle is removed for the test.
3. Measures aimed at mobilizing and removing secretions, such as chest physical therapy and intermittent positive pressure breathing (IPPB) treatments, should be performed before the tests if they are a usual part of the patient's

regimen. However, IPPB treatment should be given with saline solution only. Bronchodilators should be withheld so that the tests reflect the usual status of the patient.

4. The pulmonary function laboratory should be notified if the patient is receiving any medications affecting respiratory function. Furthermore, the time of the previous dose should be reported. This information is necessary to clarify the results of the examination.

AFTERCARE   None.

Bibliography

Ballenger, J. J. *Diseases of the Nose, Throat and Ear* (11th ed.). Philadelphia: Lea & Febiger, 1969.

Comroe, J. H., et al. *The Lung.* Chicago: Year Book, 1962.

DeWeese, D. D., and Saunders, W. H. *Textbook of Otolaryngology* (4th ed.). St. Louis: Mosby, 1973.

Foley, M. F. Pulmonary function testing. *Am. J. Nurs.* 7:1134, 1971.

Fraser, R. G., and Paré, J. A. P. *Diagnosis of Diseases of the Chest.* Philadelphia: Saunders, 1970.

Gibbon, J. H., Sabiston, D. C., Jr., and Spencer, F. C. *Surgery of the Chest* (2d ed.). Philadelphia: Saunders, 1969.

Rosenow, E. C., III, and Hughes, R. W., Jr. Progress in bronchoesophageal endoscopy. *Surg. Clin. North Am.* 53:775, 1973.

Schwaber, J. R. Evaluation of respiratory status in surgical patients. *Surg. Clin. North Am.* 50:637, 1970.

Wade, J. F. *Respiratory Nursing Care.* St. Louis: Mosby, 1973.

Bibliography

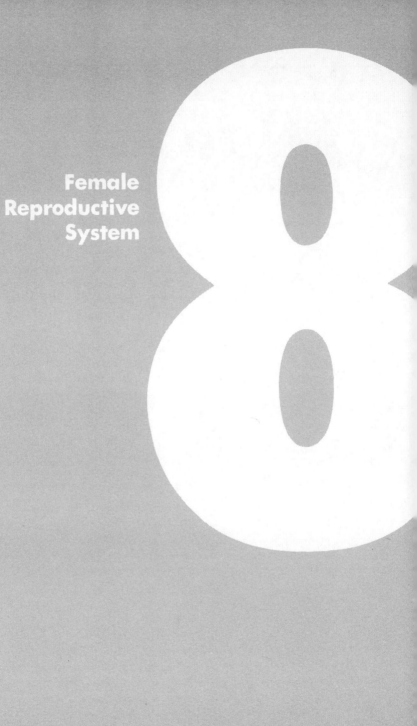

Female
Reproductive
System

8

Mammography

PURPOSE   Roentgenographic visualization of the breast without the use of contrast material.

Besides determining whether a palpable lesion is benign or malignant, mammography is a means of demonstrating breast cancer before objective signs become evident.

TIME   Twenty to 30 minutes.

LOCATION   Radiology department.

PERSONNEL   Technician.

EQUIPMENT   X-ray equipment, including a small platform on which to place the breast and a cone-shaped apparatus through which the x-ray beam is projected.

TECHNIQUE   Two views of each breast are routinely obtained, the craniocaudad and the mediolateral (Fig. 8-1). A third film is sometimes made of the axillary area, with positioning similar to that for the mediolateral view.

The accuracy of the films depends on proper positioning. The breast must be placed on the film holder in a way that reduces wrinkles, air pockets, or skin folds. Frequent repositioning may extend examination time. The patient must understand that this is done in an effort to obtain the clearest films.

PREPARATION   The patient must remove all garments above the waist. Any bandage or adhesive tape must also be removed. If tape has been used the skin must be cleansed prior to the examination. The patient must refrain from using powder, deodorant, perfume, or creams the day of the examination. Any of these items may cause extraneous shadows to appear on the films.

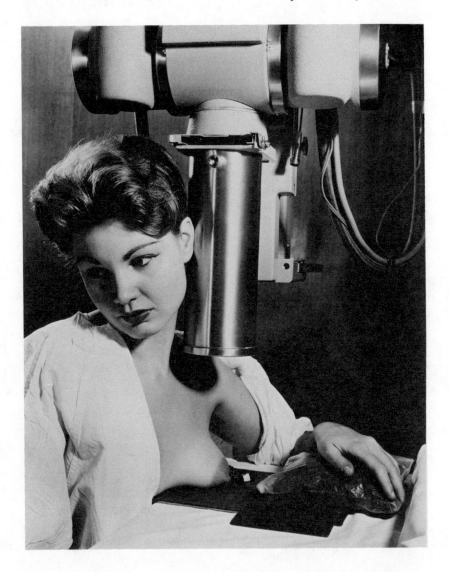

A

Figure 8-1. Patient positioning for mammography. **A.** Position for craniocaudad view. **B.** Position for mediolateral view. (From Egan, R. L., *Mammography*, 2nd Ed., 1972. Courtesy of Charles C Thomas, Publisher, Springfield, Illinois.)

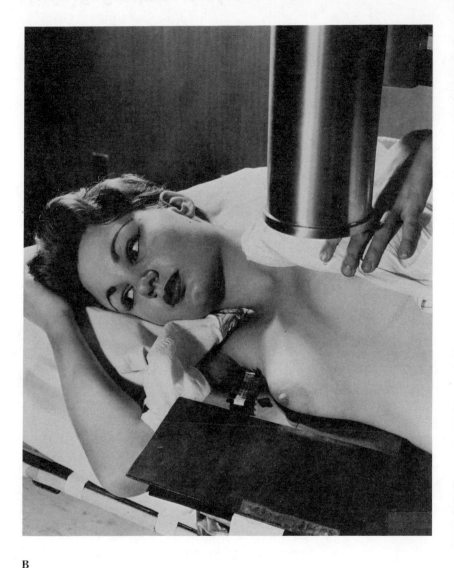

B

| PATIENT SENSATIONS | 1. As cancer of the breast is a common fear among women, a procedure performed to validate or negate this possibility is bound to be associated with some degree of fear. |
| | 2. Exposure of the breasts causes some women embarrassment and discomfort. |

AFTERCARE   None.

Hysterosalpingography

PURPOSE
Roentgenographic visualization of the uterus and fallopian tubes.

This procedure is performed primarily to investigate female infertility. It documents the presence or absence of tubal patency.

TIME
Thirty minutes to 1 hour.

LOCATION
Radiology department.

PERSONNEL
Radiologist/gynecologist and technician.

EQUIPMENT
X-ray table with stirrups, fluoroscopy unit, and overhead x-ray apparatus.

TECHNIQUE
The patient is placed on the x-ray table in the lithotomy position. A speculum is inserted into the vagina and a cannula is passed through to the uterine cervix. Under fluoroscopic guidance the contrast material is injected. Spot films are made until the uterus and tubes have been completely opacified. The cannula and speculum are then withdrawn. Further filming is determined by the type of contrast medium utilized.

1. If an oily contrast material such as Lipiodol is used, a film is obtained 24 hours after injection. Contrast material in the peritoneal cavity is indicative of tubal patency.
2. When a water-soluble agent such as Salpix is used, the contrast medium should be seen in the peritoneal cavity within 15 minutes if the tubes are patent. Delayed films may be taken until peritoneal spill is evidenced. Because of the danger of oil embolization and adhesions resulting from the use of Lipiodol, a water-soluble agent is more frequently used.

PREPARATION 1. The patient may be required to remain fasting for several hours before the test. A mild cathartic is taken the evening before the procedure and the patient is instructed to void immediately before the examination begins. These measures are directed toward preventing extraneous shadows from obscuring the anatomy involved.

2. Some gynecologists prefer to perform this procedure early in the menstrual cycle to avoid disrupting a possible pregnancy and because the procedure may in itself remove an occlusion of the fallopian tubes, thus allowing pregnancy to take place. During this early phase, however, pain and anxiety may cause cornual contractions which will occlude the tubes. A relaxant such as Diazepam may be given to overcome this. Other gynecologists prefer to perform the test just before menses, as the cornua are relaxed and cannot block the flow of contrast material. When an oil-based medium is used, the procedure is performed in the middle of the menstrual cycle when uterine vascularity is reduced. The danger of oil emboli, the primary complication of the procedure when using this type of contrast agent, is thereby minimized.

PATIENT SENSATIONS 1. The patient undergoing this procedure is usually a young woman who has been unable to conceive. Investigating the causes of sterility is bound to be associated with considerable anxiety. Its intensity will be determined by many factors, including her relationship with the man involved, the value she places on the mother role, and any previous testing she has experienced.

2. The amount and intensity of discomfort or pain vary with the patency of the fallopian tubes and the kind of contrast material that is employed. The injection of contrast material into an occluded tube can cause very severe pain persisting for several hours. When a water-soluble agent is utilized, pain is experienced as it spills into the peritoneal cavity, but usually lasts for only a few minutes.

AFTERCARE 1. Coitus may be resumed immediately.

2. If an oil-base medium was used, evidence of oil emboli should be reported. This includes chills, low-grade fever, dyspnea, cough, pleuritic pain, cyanosis, or a combination of these signs.

Amniocentesis

PURPOSE   Removal of amniotic fluid for laboratory analysis.

During the fourth or fifth month of pregnancy amniocentesis is done to detect genetic abnormalities in the fetus. In the seventh or eighth month it is performed to evaluate fetal maturity and to determine chances of survival if delivery is necessary at that time.

TIME   Ten minutes.

LOCATION   Examination room, bedside, or physician's office.

PERSONNEL   Physician (obstetrician) and assistant.

PREPARATION 1. This procedure is often preceded by ultrasonography which permits localization of the placenta, thereby minimizing fetal risk.
2. Voiding immediately before the procedure will prevent inadvertent puncture of a distended bladder.
3. Coughing, talking, and laughing should be minimized in order to limit movement of the abdomen.

TECHNIQUE 1. If the examination is performed in the early part of pregnancy, the patient is placed in a dorsal semirecumbent position, thus relaxing the abdominal musculature. If the procedure is done late in the pregnancy, the position is one of slight Trendelenburg, thereby raising the fetus out of the pelvis.
2. The abdomen is cleansed with an antiseptic solution, the puncture site infiltrated with a local anesthetic, and the adjacent areas covered with sterile drapes.
3. A needle with stylet is introduced into the uterus suprapubically. After the stylet is withdrawn, a syringe is attached to the needle and a sample of the amniotic fluid aspirated.

4. The needle is removed and the puncture site covered with a Band-Aid.
5. When the examination is performed in the latter part of pregnancy, the fetal heart rate is checked before and after the procedure.

PATIENT SENSATIONS   Because local anesthesia is employed, no pain should be experienced except that of a burning sensation as the area is infiltrated.

AFTERCARE   The presence of fever, chills, pain, or drainage from the puncture site or the vagina should be reported immediately.

Bibliography

Avnet, N. L., and Elkin, M.   Hysterosalpingography.   *Radiol. Clin. North Am.*
   5:105, 1967.
Egan, R. L.   *Mammography* (2d ed.).   Springfield, Ill.: Thomas, 1972.
Egan, R. L.   Mammography.   *Am. J. Nurs.* 66:108, 1966.
Nitowsky, H. N.   Prenatal diagnosis of genetic abnormality.   *Am. J. Nurs.*
   71:1551, 1971.
Te Linde, R. W., and Mattingly, R. F.   *Operative Gynecology* (4th ed.).
   Philadelphia: Lippincott, 1970.
Wolfe, J. N.   Mammography.   *Radiol. Clin. North Am.* 12:189, 1974.

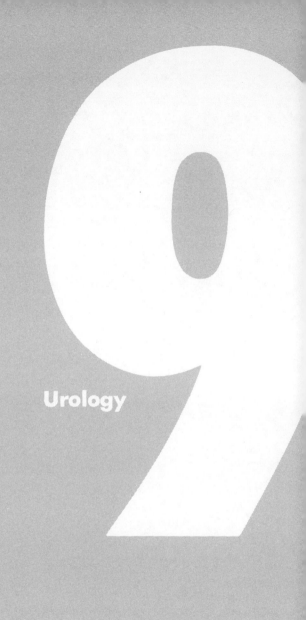

Urology

Excretory Urography
(Intravenous Pyelography [IVP])

PURPOSE   Roentgenographic visualization of the renal parenchyma,
               calices, and pelves and the ureters and bladder.

TIME   Forty-five minutes.

LOCATION   Radiology department.

PERSONNEL   Radiologist to inject the contrast material; technician to
               perform the remainder of the procedure.

EQUIPMENT   Routine x-ray table, overhead x-ray apparatus, and tomo-
               graphic equipment.

TECHNIQUE   With the patient in a supine position, a scout film is taken.
               The radiologist injects a small amount of the contrast medium
               into an antecubital vein. If no hypersensitivity reaction
               occurs within 3 minutes, the remainder is injected. Three
               postinjection films are obtained, usually at intervals of 5, 10,
               and 15 minutes. This time sequence varies with the institu-
               tion.
                   After the 5-minute film, some form of compression device
               is usually placed around the lower abdomen to retain the
               contrast medium in the upper urinary tract. After the 10-
               minute film, the compression is removed and the next
               exposure is made as the contrast agent moves into the lower
               ureters and bladder.
                   Each film is processed and inspected immediately. In-
               spection serves the radiologist as a guide to what additional
               views are needed. These may include:
               1. A film exposed after the patient voids to demonstrate
                  mucosal abnormalities and the presence or absence of
                  residual urine.

2. Tomographic cuts for the clarification of particular
   structures.
3. Delayed films (several hours after the examination) for
   adequate opacification if renal function is impaired or if
   there is stasis in the upper part of the urinary tract, as in
   ureteral obstruction.

The following are modifications of the standard technique :

1. Drip infusion IVP
   A large volume of contrast material mixed with 5% dextrose
   in water or normal saline solution is infused rapidly to
   achieve denser opacification. This variation is usually
   done on patients in whom the standard technique has
   failed to yield sufficient diagnostic information. It may
   also be done when other data such as an elevated BUN
   level indicate that concentration of the contrast medium
   will be poor using the standard technique.
2. Rapid-sequence method for hypertension
   The sequence of filming is altered when renal artery
   stenosis is suspected as the causative factor of hypertension.
   Immediately after injection, films are exposed at 1-minute
   intervals for 5 minutes. Information is provided on the
   exact time of excretion of the contrast material by each
   kidney, and any differences between the two can be
   detected. From this point the examination continues
   as for standard urography.

   In the investigation of hypertension, a washout film
   may be obtained. Diuresis is induced by administering
   an osmotic diuretic such as urea or mannitol. While the
   normal collecting system becomes less radiopaque as the
   contrast medium is diluted, the kidney that is ischemic
   secondary to renal artery stenosis remains unchanged.
3. Nephrotomography
   Nephrotomograms are serial tomographic cuts obtained
   with the renal parenchyma opacified. Nephrotomography
   may be performed as a separate procedure or done during
   standard urography. It is performed primarily to differentiate whether a kidney mass is a cyst or a solid tumor.
   Tomograms are obtained both before the injection of the
   contrast agent to determine the planes which maximize
   demonstration of the lesion, and after the contrast has

opacified the renal parenchyma and started filling the calices and renal pelves. Additional exposures are made as needed at different depths through the kidney to discern the thickness of the wall of the mass and the nature of the interior of the mass.

PREPARATION
1. A strong cathartic is administered in the late afternoon prior to the examination. Intestinal gas and feces must be removed so that details will not be obscured on the films.
2. The patient is permitted only a light dinner and should remain NPO from midnight preceding the examination. The moderate dehydration thus achieved permits concentration of the contrast material. When a drip infusion IVP is to be performed, this partial dehydration is not necessary.
3. The patient voids immediately before the procedure. A full bladder will dilute the contrast material entering it, thereby reducing opacification of this structure.
4. The patient should be forewarned of the time intervals between films to avoid anxiety at being left alone for extended periods of time between pictures.

PATIENT SENSATIONS
1. The patient will experience the pain associated with venipuncture.
2. Depending on the contrast agent employed, the patient may experience transitory pain in the arm in which the injection is given.
3. Some common side-effects result from the contrast material. These include a generalized feeling of warmth, nausea, vomiting, and a metallic taste in the mouth. More severe and potentially fatal reactions include anaphylaxis and cardiovascular collapse. The patient should report any unusual feeling, no matter how minimal.
4. No discomfort should be experienced from the compression belt. If any pain is felt, the technician should be informed so that the belt can be readjusted.

AFTERCARE
None. If any untoward reactions occur as a result of the contrast material, the patient or staff will be informed of any special instructions regarding the patient's care.

Cystoscopy (Cystourethroscopy)

PURPOSE   Direct visualization of the bladder, urethra, and ureteral orifices to detect abnormalities of structure and function, or as preparation for radiographic study of the upper urinary tract.

TIME   Five to 45 minutes depending on the ease with which the cystoscope is inserted, the problem for which the examination is being performed, and whether the procedure is being carried out under general, spinal, or local anesthesia.

LOCATION   Cystoscopy suite.

PERSONNEL   Urologist, anesthesiologist, nurse, and assistants. The urologist is attired as for an operative procedure.

EQUIPMENT   Cystoscope (Fig. 9-1), cystoscopy table with leg supports for assistance in maintenance of the lithotomy position.

PREPARATION 1. The patient is kept NPO if it is to be performed under general or spinal anesthesia. Preprocedural medication to enhance anesthesia induction will be administered.
2. The patient who is to be examined under local anesthesia

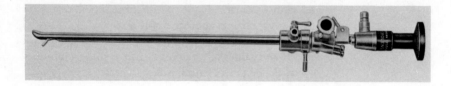

Figure 9-1. Cystoscope. (Courtesy American Cystoscope Makers, Inc., Stamford, Conn.)

may receive premedications which will permit him to remain comfortable and anxiety-free during the procedure.

TECHNIQUE

1. If general or spinal anesthesia is used, an intravenous infusion is started and a satisfactory level of anesthesia is achieved.
2. The patient is placed on the cystoscopy table in the lithotomy position. If he cannot tolerate this position, he is placed supine with his hips and knees flexed and slightly abducted. Sterile drapes are applied, leaving only the external genitalia exposed.
3. The urethral orifice and surrounding external genitalia are cleansed with an antiseptic solution. If general or spinal anesthesia has not been used, topical anesthesia will be introduced into the urethra.
4. The physician gently inserts the lubricated cystoscope into the bladder. If urethral strictures are present, dilatation may be necessary before the examination can proceed. Sterile fluid is instilled into the bladder to distend it and allow visualization.
5. Direct visual examination of the bladder, ureteral orifices, and urethra follows. Adjunctive equipment may be introduced through the basic cystoscope to improve visualization, insert ureteral catheters and radiopaque material, perform biopsies, or remove tissue, foreign bodies, or calculi.
6. Biopsy of the prostate through the perineum is sometimes performed based on what has been seen cystoscopically. After the perineum has been locally anesthetized, a small skin incision is made and the biopsy instrument inserted. Guidance to the appropriate area of the prostate is assisted by introduction of a finger into the rectum. A small piece of tissue is removed and the biopsy instrument withdrawn.
7. At the completion of the examination the cystoscope is withdrawn. If excessive instrumentation has been necessary, an indwelling catheter may be left in place to counteract ensuing edema and urinary retention.

PATIENT SENSATIONS

The patient may experience:
1. Considerable anxiety at the thought of this particular type of instrumentation.

2. Embarrassment from the position and from exposure and examination of the genitalia.
3. Dull pain or discomfort during introduction of the cysto-scope or during dilatation or biopsy if the procedure is done without general or regional anesthesia.
4. Fear of castration.
5. Fatigue and discomfort from maintaining the position. This may not be experienced until later if general or regional anesthesia was employed.
6. An uncomfortably distended bladder due to the fluid instilled to allow visualization. This will not be felt if regional or general anesthesia is used.

AFTERCARE
1. The time and amount of urinary output should be noted and recorded to ensure that the patient is not experiencing urinary retention secondary to edema.
2. Each voiding should be checked for hematuria.
3. Once the patient is alert and able to swallow, fluids should be encouraged to reduce inflammation.
4. Vital signs should be checked when the patient returns to his room and as frequently thereafter as necessary. Level of consciousness and motor or sensory level should also be evaluated if general or regional anesthesia was used.
5. The appearance of chills and fever, as late as 24 hours after instrumentation, may be indicative of urinary sepsis.

Retrograde Urography (Pyelography)

PURPOSE Roentgenographic visualization of the renal pelves, renal calices, and ureters to detect structural and functional abnormalities when:
1. Excretory urography is contraindicated, e.g., in the case of renal insufficiency or multiple myeloma,
2. Excretory urography has not provided adequate information owing to poor renal excretory function, or
3. An allergy to contrast material is known to exist.

The contrast material is injected directly into the ureteral catheters and not into the vascular system. Thus problems arising from its absorption and renal excretion are reduced.

TIME Thirty to 45 minutes.

LOCATION Cystoscopy suite or radiology department.

PERSONNEL Urologist, assistants, and anesthesiologist (if anesthesia is to be used).

EQUIPMENT As for cystoscopy (see page 184), plus ureteral catheters, tilting x-ray table with stirrups, and fluoroscopy unit or overhead x-ray apparatus, or both.

PREPARATION
1. Measures must be taken to clear the bowel of all gas and feces as these will cause obscuring shadows on the x-ray films.
2. The patient remains NPO before the procedure if general or spinal anesthesia is to be used.
3. Premedications will be prescribed according to whether the examination is to be performed under local or general anesthesia.
4. An intravenous infusion may be started the night before retrograde urography to ensure good urinary output if

bilateral renal urine specimens are to be obtained during the procedure for acid-fast bacillus culture.

TECHNIQUE

1. With patient in the lithotomy position, a cystoscopic examination is performed under local, regional, or general anesthesia.
2. One or more ureteral catheters are then introduced through the cystoscope.
3. Catheter placement is verified by fluoroscopy or an over-head radiograph. A small amount of contrast material is injected, usually under fluoroscopic guidance, into the ureteral catheters. If filling of the ureters and renal pelves and calices is incomplete, the patient may be tilted into the Trendelenburg position, more contrast material injected, and more films taken.
4. Once adequate filling has been achieved, anteroposterior, oblique, and lateral films are exposed.
5. The patient is then positioned semiupright on the tilting table and radiographs are taken as the catheters are with-drawn. These films will demonstrate the ureters as the contrast material flows downward. The cystoscope usually remains in position throughout the procedure.
6. Delayed films at 15 minutes are exposed to verify excre-tion of the contrast material. If complete excretion has not taken place, further films may be necessary after another waiting period. These films demonstrate the presence, location, and degree of an obstruction.
7. One ureteral catheter may be left in place in cases of ureteral obstruction until adequate postprocedural urinary output has been established. This catheter is usually secured to an indwelling bladder catheter and drainage apparatus.

PATIENT
SENSATIONS

1. Refer to the section on cystoscopy.
2. Severe renal colic and costovertebral pain persisting for several days may be experienced if too much contrast material is inadvertently injected into the renal capsule. This pain may not be felt until the effects of the regional or general anesthesia have dissipated.

3. Too large an amount of contrast material may also cause pyelotubular backflow into the systemic circulation, with the possibility of anaphylaxis.

4. Passage of both the cystoscope and the ureteral catheters may be painful if done under local anesthesia. The pain is described by the patients as dull and uncomfortable. Discomfort may be aggravated by the primary diagnosis, e.g., strictures.

AFTERCARE

1. Patients who have received general anesthesia may go to the recovery room before returning to the unit.

2. Instrumentation of the urinary tract usually causes some degree of irritation and edema which may lead to hematuria and temporary oliguria or anuria. Urinary output should be monitored by noting time and amount, as well as the presence and degree of hematuria for each specimen.

3. The patient should be observed for signs of urinary sepsis secondary to instrumentation.

4. If a ureteral catheter is left in place attached to an indwelling urethral catheter, the amount and character of the drainage from each should be noted separately. Failure of the ureteral catheter to drain should be reported immediately. Great care should be taken not to dislodge the ureteral catheter.

Voiding Cystourethrography (VCU)

PURPOSE   Roentgenographic visualization of the bladder, bladder neck, and urethra during micturition.

Abnormalities related to the lower portion of the urinary tract such as urethral obstruction and bladder diverticula may thus be evaluated and vesicoureteral reflux demonstrated.

TIME   Fifteen minutes.

LOCATION   Radiology department.

PERSONNEL   Radiologist and technician.

EQUIPMENT   X-ray table, overhead x-ray apparatus or fluoroscopy unit, and catheters.

PREPARATION   None.

TECHNIQUE
1. A urethral catheter is introduced into the bladder. The urine is drained, and contrast material is introduced, usually under fluoroscopic guidance, in sufficient quantities to cause distension and the urge to void.
2. The catheter is removed.
3. Films are taken as the patient voids and again on completion of voiding to check for vesicoureteral reflux, to visualize the anatomy of the urethra, and to determine if any residual urine remains within the bladder after voiding.

PATIENT SENSATIONS
1. The patient often feels embarrassed and inhibited at being asked to void on demand in the presence of others.
2. There should be little discomfort except for the sensation of distension and the urge to void as the bladder is filled with the contrast material.

AFTERCARE   None.

Retrograde Urethrography

PURPOSE   Roentgenographic visualization of the anterior portion of the urethra. (The posterior portion of the urethra is visualized to best advantage during voiding cystourethrography.)

TIME   Twenty minutes.

LOCATION   Radiology department.

PERSONNEL   Radiologist and technician.

EQUIPMENT   X-ray table, fluoroscopy unit or overhead x-ray apparatus, and Brodney clamp or double-ballooned catheter.

PREPARATION   None.

TECHNIQUE   1. The patient is placed in a supine position on the x-ray table.
2. In the male patient, the contrast material is instilled using the Brodney clamp, an instrument designed specifically for retrograde urethrography (Fig. 9-2). The tiny jaws of the clamp are attached to the junction of the glans and the shaft of the penis. The other end of the clamp accommodates a syringe that contains the contrast material. The Brodney clamp therefore serves two purposes. It aligns the urethra in such a way that no extraneous shadows will appear on the films since its structure does not cover any part of the penis, and it allows for injection of the contrast material. The contrast medium frequently is injected under fluoroscopic guidance and appropriate spot films are taken. Alternatively, overhead films may be obtained in lateral or oblique projections following injection of the contrast material.

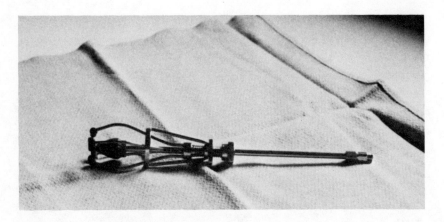

Figure 9-2. The Brodney clamp is used in male patients to instill contrast material for retrograde urethrography.

3. The female urethra is studied by inserting a double-ballooned catheter into the bladder. The first balloon is inflated in the bladder, the second inflated against the external urinary meatus. The contrast material is injected. It enters the urethra through a small hole located in the section of the catheter between the two balloons. Spot films or overhead anteroposterior and oblique films are obtained.

PATIENT SENSATIONS Moderate discomfort may be experienced if the urethra is distended by the contrast material. The patient should immediately inform the physician of such discomfort so that injection may be discontinued.

Male patients may fear castration with application of the Brodney clamp.

AFTERCARE The patient should be observed closely for the onset of chills or fever. Too large an amount or too forceful an injection of the contrast material into the urethra may cause its extravasation along with any urethral contaminants into the circulatory system.

Cystometry

PURPOSE   Evaluation of intravesical pressure and thermal sensation.
This procedure is frequently performed when evidence
of neurological dysfunction of the bladder exists.

TIME   Thirty minutes to 1 hour.

LOCATION   Urological diagnostic suite.

PERSONNEL   Physician, nurse, or technician.

EQUIPMENT   Foley catheter and associated equipment, and cystometer
(Fig. 9-3).

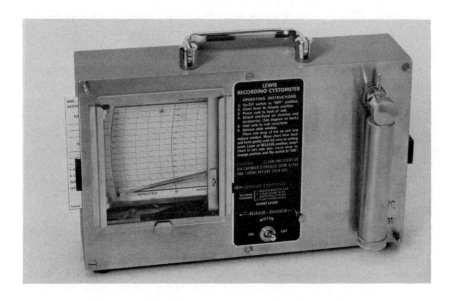

Figure 9-3. Lewis cystometer. (Courtesy American Cystoscope Makers, Inc.,
Stamford, Conn.)

TECHNIQUE
1. A Foley catheter is inserted. Consistency of catheter size within an institution is necessary, as differences in lumen size will affect pressure readings, making it difficult to establish a standard baseline for the procedure. This will affect accurate interpretation of the recording.
2. The examination is performed with the patient in a supine position.
3. Thermal sensation is evaluated by the consecutive introduction into the bladder of relatively small amounts of hot and cold sterile fluid. In each case, the patient is asked to tell the examiner what temperature, if any, is experienced during the irrigation. The fluid is either aspirated or permitted to drain from the catheter.
4. A 1000-ml bottle of normal saline solution is connected to the cystometer and the catheter. The fluid is allowed to flow into the bladder at a standard rate and the pressures within the bladder are graphically measured and recorded by the cystometer. The patient is asked to report such sensations as flushing, sweating, nausea, pain, feeling of bladder fullness, and an overwhelming urge to void. These sensations are related to the neurological innervation of the bladder and sphincters. Correlations are made between the volume of fluid instilled and the time that the particular sensation is noted.
5. Fluid is continuously instilled until the patient feels that he is unable to inhibit voiding any longer and voids involuntarily around the catheter.
6. The patient should be warned not to strain at any point, as this will increase intraabdominal and intravesical pressure, thereby altering cystometric readings.
7. Any residual fluid is withdrawn and measured.
8. Pharmacological agents may be administered during cystometry. Bethanechol chloride (Urecholine) is used to evaluate the response of an atonic bladder to parasympathomimetic action. Atropine or a similar parasympatholytic agent is given to assess its inhibiting effect on a hyperactive bladder. This additional feature of the examination will extend the time required for cystometry.

PREPARATION
1. If this procedure is performed on an inpatient basis, the Foley catheter may be inserted before the patient leaves the unit for the examination.
2. Because this procedure is often done on patients with a neurological deficit, which may include a motor component, transfer to the examination table may be difficult. If this is the case, the patient should be transported on a stretcher. The procedure may then be performed without the necessity of moving the patient to the examining table.
3. Patients sometimes confuse cystometry with cystography, a radiological procedure. The differences should be clarified so that the patient comprehends the benignity of a cystometrogram.

PATIENT SENSATIONS
1. The patient should be forewarned of the sense of bladder fullness, the overwhelming urge to void, and the subsequent involuntary voiding around the catheter. It should be emphasized that these are normal and expected occurrences.
2. There may be a sensation of air in the bladder when it is emptied by aspiration.

AFTERCARE
None.

Electronic Evaluation of Urinary Flow Rate

PURPOSE   Evaluation of urethral obstruction by measuring the force of a voided stream of urine.

TIME   Ten to 15 minutes.

LOCATION   A small enclosed area within the urological diagnostic suite.

PERSONNEL   Nurse or technician.

EQUIPMENT   Elevated commodelike chair, and funnel and graduated glass cylinder attached to an electronic pressure-recording device which writes out a line graph of pressures throughout voiding (Fig. 9-4).

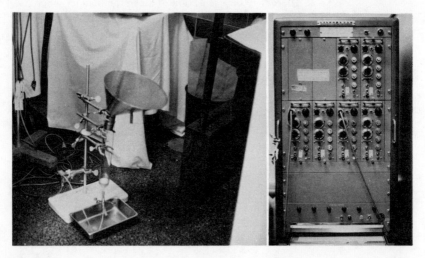

A   B

Figure 9-4.   Equipment used for electronic evaluation of urinary flow rate. **A.** Funnel and cylindrical collecting device. **B.** Electronic pressure-recording device.

TECHNIQUE
1. The patient is asked to void into the glass cylinder which is made accessible by attaching a wide-mouth funnel to it. A male patient may stand and void directly into the funnel; a woman is seated on the raised chair and the collecting device placed directly beneath the hole in the chair's seat.
2. Pressures are measured and recorded by the electronic console throughout voiding. The amount of urine and duration of voiding are also noted.
3. Privacy is secured by having the patient void in an enclosed area.

PREPARATION
In a 2- to 4-hour period before the scheduled time of the test, the patient is asked to drink at least a quart of any type of fluid. Intake may be spread out over that period of time. The patient should arrive for the test with a distended feeling and an urge to void. He should not void during this "loading" period.

PATIENT SENSATIONS
It may be inhibiting and embarrassing to be asked to void on demand. The patient should know that he will not be under direct observation even though there will be someone in the diagnostic suite. Assurance should be given that such feelings are common and that every measure will be made to ensure privacy during the test.

AFTERCARE
None.

Renal Biopsy

PURPOSE Removal of a minute portion of renal tissue for histological examination.

TIME Fifteen minutes.

LOCATION Urological diagnostic suite or treatment room.

PERSONNEL Physician (usually a nephrologist) and assistant.

EQUIPMENT Biopsy needle and fixative for tissue specimens.

PREPARATION
1. A complete hematological evaluation is done, as bleeding is a major complication of biopsy.
2. Blood is typed and cross matched and held on call.
3. A plain film of the abdomen or an excretory urogram is taken to localize the kidney.
4. Premedication with a sedative and an analgesic is administered to ensure that the patient will be comfortable, calm, and able to follow directions during the procedure.

TECHNIQUE
1. The patient is placed in a prone position with pillows beneath the abdomen to bring the kidneys closer to the surface of the back.
2. The area is cleansed with an antiseptic solution, sterilely draped, and infiltrated with a local anesthetic. The right kidney is usually chosen to avoid puncture of the spleen and great vessels, which lie on the left side.
3. The patient is instructed to take a deep breath and hold it as the biopsy needle is introduced and advanced. Once the needle is in the kidney, the patient is instructed to breathe normally.
4. After the biopsy specimen has been obtained, the needle is removed and firm pressure applied to the site.

PATIENT SENSATIONS

1. There will be a momentary stinging sensation as the local anesthetic is injected, then a feeling of numbness.
2. The patient may feel pressure as the biopsy needle is introduced and advanced but should feel no pain.
3. Severe ureteral colic may be felt after the biopsy if bleeding has occurred and a clot is being passed.

AFTERCARE

Bleeding is the major complication of renal biopsy. Most patients will have microscopic hematuria; a few will have gross hematuria. To prevent the possibility of hemorrhage the patient is maintained on bed rest for 24 hours following the procedure and increased intake of fluids is encouraged. Vital signs are monitored and hematocrit values determined frequently.

Bibliography

Campbell, M. F., and Harrison, J. H. *Urology* (3d ed.). Philadelphia: Saunders, 1970.

Emmett, J. L., and Witten, D. M. *Clinical Urography: An Atlas and Textbook of Roentgenologic Diagnosis.* Philadelphia: Saunders, 1971.

Pollack, H. M. *Radiologic Examination of the Urinary Tract.* New York: Harper & Row, 1971.

Smith, D. R. *General Urology* (7th ed.). Los Altos, Calif.: Lange, 1972.

10

Radioisotope
Scanning

General Aspects

Nuclear medicine, which employs radioisotopes to study and treat disease, is a rapidly developing field, especially in the area of diagnostic procedures. This chapter will describe some of the diagnostic studies most commonly performed. As there are several elements common to all of these procedures, they will be discussed in this introduction rather than with each procedure.

RADIO-PHARMA-CEUTICALS (TRACERS)

A radiopharmaceutical is a chemical compound containing a minute amount of a radioisotope. Gamma rays, one of several different types of radiation, are emitted by the radioisotope and registered by the scanning instrument.

The radiopharmaceutical is chosen because of its selective localization in a particular organ or tissue. Some radiopharmaceuticals localize in normal tissue, others in abnormal tissue. Other factors involved in the choice include maintenance of the lowest possible level of radiation dosage to the patient, and the production and storage facilities within the institution. Examples of commonly used radiopharmaceuticals are iodine 131 (^{131}I), technetium 99m pertechnetate (^{99m}Tc pertechnetate), radioiodinated serum albumin (^{131}RISA), and mercury 197 chlormerodrin (^{197}Hg chlormerodrin).

SCANNING EQUIPMENT

There are two basic types of detectors in common use, the rectilinear scanner and the gamma camera. Both may be likened to highly refined types of Geiger counter, a device that detects emissions from a radioactive source and converts them into signals which can be recorded and interpreted.

The rectilinear scanner (Fig. 10-1) was developed first. It has a very small field of view, which necessitates its moving back and forth either vertically or horizontally at a predetermined

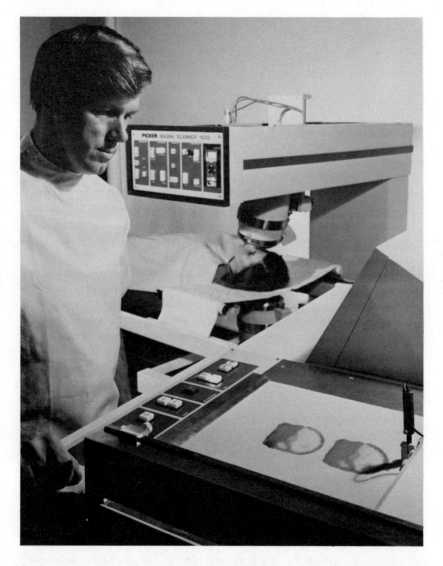

Figure 10-1. Picker Magna Scanner 1000 (rectilinear scanner) with patient having brain scan. Imaging device travels back and forth over the area to be scanned. Results are displayed on x-ray film, paper, or a screen. (Courtesy Picker Corporation, Cleveland, Ohio.)

distance and rate across the organ to be scanned until the entire area has been covered. It operates by converting radiation emissions into electrical pulses which can be counted. These counts are usually recorded as dots on x-ray film or paper. Sometimes the count is also visualized on an oscilloscope, enabling the technician to adjust the position of either the patient or the machine. The information may also be simultaneously stored in a computer data bank for future retrieval.

A more recent imaging device is the gamma camera (Fig. 10-2). Its much larger field of vision obviates the need for motion and frequently permits imaging to be performed more quickly than when a rectilinear scanner is used. It can be appropriately positioned next to the patient and with few exceptions encompasses the entire area to be scanned.

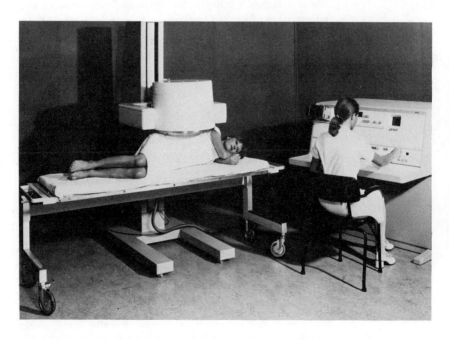

Figure 10-2. Scintillation gamma camera allows continuous imaging of entire area under study. Results are viewed on an oscilloscope. (Courtesy Philips Medical Systems, Inc., Shelton, Conn.)

The camera's imaging devices permit continuous visualization of the accumulation and distribution of the radiopharmaceutical. This is viewed on an oscilloscope screen. Scintiphotographs (pictures) of the image are taken with a camera at preset intervals of time. These time periods are related to the moment when a predetermined number of counts is reached. Although the gamma camera produces an image without actually scanning, the term *scan* is still in common use and will be used here to refer to both types of instruments.

Since most scans are performed with the patient in some variation of a horizontal position, the room will contain, in addition to the scanning equipment, a stretcher or table similar to that used for radiological procedures.

TIME The duration of a scan and the amount of time between administration of the radiopharmaceutical and the start of the scan will be affected by three factors: (1) the radiopharmaceutical chosen, (2) the type of scanning device used, and (3) the speed with which the radiation emission builds up to a countable level.

LOCATION These procedures may be performed in either a radiology or a nuclear medicine department.

PERSONNEL There will always be a trained nuclear medicine technician present with the patient during the procedure. However, it is usually the physician trained in nuclear medicine who administers the radiopharmaceutical. A nurse is not usually present but may accompany the patient should his particular illness warrant it.

PREPARATION Patients often have more questions concerning the radiation hazards of scanning than of other radiology procedures. It may seem more dangerous since the radioisotope must be ingested or injected. In addition some patients believe that the scanner emits radiation like an x-ray machine. In most scans the dose of radiation received is less than, or at most equal to, that received during the production of a single x-ray film. Any danger to the patient from a radiopharmaceutical is always weighed very carefully against the potential benefits of the procedure. At times performance of a scan may obviate the need for a more difficult and dangerous procedure, e.g., angiography. It should be stressed that radiopharmaceuticals are given in such small amounts that there is no danger of sterility. Furthermore, it should be pointed out that a scanning device is a benign instrument which receives rather than emits radiation.

Preparation sometimes includes the use of a nonradioactive pharmaceutical called a *blocking agent*. It is taken up by organs other than the one under study. This prevents them from receiving unnecessary radiation from the circulating radiopharmaceutical and ensures that all the radiopharmaceutical goes to the organ being studied. If the radiopharmaceutical were taken up by adjacent organs, the scan image would be obscured by intervening radiation. The most common blocking agents are listed below. (1) Lugol's solution is an oral preparation containing iodine which is administered to an individual receiving an iodine radioisotope for any organ scan except that of the thyroid. Its action is in blocking uptake of isotope by the thyroid. Since it has an unpleasant taste and stains the teeth, it is best administered in juice and through a straw. The commencement and duration of administration as well as dosage will vary with the institution and the type of scan to be performed. (2) Potassium perchlorate is often given to individuals who are allergic to iodine. It is administered orally and its taste has been compared to that of stale water. It is useful in brain scanning as it is taken up by the salivary glands and the choroid plexus of the lateral cerebral ventricles. These organs might otherwise obscure areas of abnormal uptake and make interpretation of the brain scan difficult or inaccurate. It can be used for other types of scans but this decision depends on whether the physician considers its utilization of value in improving the clarity and precision of imaging. (3) Meralluride or sodium mercaptomerin is usually administered intramuscularly prior to a scan in which the radiopharmaceutical is ^{197}Hg chlormerodrin. It is given to block uptake of isotope by the kidneys.

A patient who is allergic to iodine and is therefore unable

to tolerate the radioiodinated contrast mediums used in many radiological studies may safely undergo a scanning procedure. Should the use of ^{131}I be necessary, the amount given is so minute as to make the possibility of an allergic reaction extremely unlikely. However, the most frequently used blocking agent for ^{131}I is Lugol's solution, an iodine preparation, and therefore to be avoided. Other blocking agents free of iodine are available, or another radiopharmaceutical may be given.

It is important that the patient understand the necessity of maintaining each position in which he is placed so as to obtain as accurate an image as possible. He should be encouraged to express any sensations of discomfort so that a more comfortable position may be found before each part of the scan begins.

The patient should be forewarned that more than one scan or type of scan may be necessary and is not automatically a sign of a serious disorder.

All scans may be performed on either an inpatient or an outpatient basis.

PATIENT
SENSATIONS

Beyond the mild transitory pain of venipuncture and the discomfort of maintaining a possibly awkward position for an extended period of time, there should be no discomfort specifically associated with a scan. However, it should always be kept in mind that pain, difficulty in breathing, and restlessness, which may interfere with maintenance of position and jeopardize the success of the procedure, may be among the signs and symptoms which have necessitated the scan. When any of these factors is present, it should be evaluated and appropriate measures taken to ensure maximum patient comfort and cooperation.

A rectilinear scanner will produce a soft, continuous, irregular clicking noise as it registers the radiation emissions.

AFTERCARE

Rarely is physical aftercare necessary. When specific actions are required, they will be enumerated in the units that follow.

Dynamic Blood Flow Studies (Radionuclide Angiography)

PURPOSE   To evaluate the patency and function of major blood vessels and the blood supply of an organ or of any lesions within it.

TIME   One minute.

PREPARATION   A blocking agent may be given depending on the radiopharmaceutical chosen.

TECHNIQUE   The patient is positioned according to the organ to be studied. Scanning with a gamma camera begins immediately after injection of the radiopharmaceutical. Serial scintiphotographs are taken at preset intervals of 2 to 3 seconds. Radionuclide angiography may be followed by a static scan of the same organ.

PATIENT SENSATIONS   The gamma camera is positioned very close to the area to be studied. If cerebral blood flow is being evaluated, the patient may experience claustrophobic feelings at having such a large, heavy instrument looming directly above his face.

Bone Scan

PURPOSE
1. To detect bone disease, including primary and metastatic bone cancer.
2. To determine portals of entry for radiotherapy.
3. To evaluate progress of a disease or efficacy of management.

TIME
One and one-half to 2 hours.

TECHNIQUE
^{99m}Tc diphosphonate and polyphosphate are the tracers of choice owing to their greater safety, ease of use, and diagnostic range. Their bone-seeking mechanism is not fully understood, but their effectiveness and greater margin of radiation safety in contrast to the previously used strontium and fluorine make them desirable.

The radiopharmaceutical is injected intravenously 3 hours before the scan is begun. During the interim the hospitalized patient may return to his room. Just before the scan he will be asked to void.

Positioning will be determined by the area to be scanned, but will usually be supine. If a gamma camera is used, the patient's position will be changed approximately every 4 minutes according to the views considered necessary.

Reference points of special interest, such as areas of pain, may be marked by the physician with a skin pencil for later correlation of the scan with x-ray films. When posterior films are necessary, the patient is positioned on his abdomen. This position is often extremely uncomfortable for an individual who is usually already plagued by pain.

Although neoplastic or metastatic processes are likely to be recognized 3 to 6 months earlier on scans than on x-ray films, many other diseases also appear on a scan. Therefore, x-ray films must be taken of suspect areas within 1 to 2 weeks of the scan to provide comparison and thus a more accurate diagnosis.

Brain Scan

PURPOSE   To determine:
1. The presence of an intracranial space-occupying lesion or vascular abnormality.
2. The nature of the lesion.
3. The response of the patient to treatment.
4. The progressive course of a diagnosed lesion.

TIME
1. Rectilinear scanner — 45 to 60 minutes
2. Gamma camera — 10 to 15 minutes

PREPARATION   A blocking agent may be given depending on the radiopharmaceutical chosen.

TECHNIQUE   At the appropriate time after receiving the radiopharmaceutical either orally or intravenously, the patient is placed in a supine position on a stretcher so that his head is directly aligned with the scanner or camera (see Fig. 10-1). Anterior, posterior, and both lateral views are taken. The patient's position may have to be changed accordingly. If special views of the posterior fossa are desired, it will be necessary to place the patient in a supine position with his head flexed forward onto his chest and a strap placed across his forehead to restrict movement.

When screening for lesions is the objective of the study, ^{99m}Tc or ^{197}Hg chlormerodrin is usually the preferred scanning agent. ^{99m}Tc has a very short physical half-life and when given intravenously permits immediate scanning. It is often preferred when there are localizing signs in the posterior fossa because of the high counts obtained with the usual quantity given.

Once an abnormality has been found, a second scan using ^{131}RISA may be performed to determine the nature of the abnormality. Scans are performed immediately after intravenous administration of ^{131}RISA, then at 24 hours and 48 hours. Tentative identification of lesions is possible because different lesions become more clearly visible at specific time intervals, e.g., arteriovenous malformations immediately after injection and metastatic lesions at 24 hours.

Dynamic radionuclide angiography may be done immediately prior to a static brain scan.

Cardiac Blood Pool Scan

PURPOSE To evaluate the size, shape, and position of the heart and great vessels.

The primary value of this procedure is in detecting pericardial effusions, but only if they are greater than 200 ml.

TIME Two to 3 minutes.

PREPARATION A blocking agent may be given depending on the radiopharmaceutical chosen.

TECHNIQUE The patient is usually placed in a supine position with the gamma camera directly above his chest. If he is orthopneic, he may be scanned in a sitting position. Scanning is begun immediately after injection of the radiopharmaceutical.

Intrathecal Scan
(Radioisotope Cisternography)

PURPOSE   Introduction of a radiopharmaceutical into the intrathecal (subarachnoid) space to:
1. Evaluate alterations in the distribution and flow of cerebrospinal fluid (CSF) and its effects on the cerebral ventricular system.
2. Identify and locate the presence of a CSF leak.

TIME
1. Ten to 15 minutes for lumbar puncture and introduction of the radioisotope
2. One- to 3-hour interval before the scan begins
3. Forty-five to 60 minutes for scanning with a rectilinear scanner
4. Ten to 15 minutes for scanning with a gamma camera
5. Up to 72 hours to obtain a series of scans

EQUIPMENT   Lumbar puncture tray (see page 15).

PREPARATION
1. A blocking agent may be given depending on the radiopharmaceutical chosen.
2. Explanation of a lumbar puncture should be included (see pages 15–19).
3. Lumbar puncture should not be performed prior to this procedure as intrathecal injection may be difficult if other punctures have been done recently. CSF may be withdrawn immediately prior to injection of the radiopharmaceutical for laboratory analysis.
4. Intrathecal scanning is usually done in conjunction with other procedures to obtain all possible information. If pneumoencephalography is among the procedures planned, scanning should precede it. If this is not possible, the institution's policy may require at least a week's hiatus before scanning may be performed.

TECHNIQUE   A lumbar puncture is performed and a syringe containing
the radiopharmaceutical agent is attached to the spinal needle.
One to 2 ml of CSF is aspirated into the syringe; the mixture
in the syringe is then reinjected into the intrathecal space.
Minimal manipulation of the needle is important during the
procedure, and spinal fluid pressure is usually not measured to
ensure an accurate reflection of the patient's normal CSF
dynamics and to minimize the possibility of extravasation
of the agent into the epidural space. Should the latter occur,
the procedure is usually terminated and rescheduled for a
later date to ensure that the radiopharmaceutical has been
completely excreted from the body and will not affect the
accuracy of the future procedure or give the patient excessive
radiation exposure.

One to 2 hours after injection scanning is begun with the
patient in a supine position. Both anterior and lateral views
are obtained. These may be accomplished simultaneously if
a dual-probe rectilinear scanner is used. When a gamma
camera is the chosen instrument, the two views are taken
serially. These same views are taken again at regular intervals
for up to 72 hours following lumbar puncture. The number
and timing are determined by departmental policy and the
diagnostic problem under investigation.

To diagnose a CSF leak, sterile cotton pledgets are placed
in the nose or ear following introduction of the radiopharmaceutical. They are collected and their radioactivity
assayed after the test period.

Once a CSF leak is verified, identification of its source is
accomplished by the administration of a larger than usual
dose of radiopharmaceutical by lumbar puncture. Afterward
the patient is placed in a supine position for approximately
3 hours to allow the tracer time to reach the brain, and to
prevent further CSF leakage.

At the end of this time, the patient is placed in a seated
position with his head down and a gamma camera placed for
a lateral view. Scanning is then begun. The patient may be
asked to perform a Valsalva maneuver to encourage leakage.
Several scintiphotographs are taken at preset intervals until
the leak is visualized. An anterior view is then obtained to
define more specifically the location of the leak.

PATIENT
SENSATIONS

1. Refer to the section on lumbar puncture.
2. The cotton pledgets in the patient's nose necessitate mouth breathing and cause a very dry mouth and in some patients a sense of not being able to breathe adequately.
3. Sitting in a head-down position may also be uncomfortable even though support is provided.

AFTERCARE

1. Refer to the section on lumbar puncture.
2. Alterations in neurological status and vital signs should be monitored carefully. Particular attention should be paid to an elevation in temperature. Aseptic meningitis is a possible complication when ^{131}I human serum albumin (RIHSA) is used. Bacterial meningitis is a complication of a CSF leak.

Liver Scan

PURPOSE   To evaluate:
1. Liver structure, i.e., size, shape, and location.
2. Liver function, e.g., biliary duct patency.

TIME
1. Liver structure scan — 30 to 45 minutes.
2. Liver function (rose bengal) scan — up to three scans of approximately 30 minutes each within 24 hours. The time intervals will vary with the institution. Sometimes an additional scan at 48 hours is required.

PREPARATION A blocking agent may be given depending on the radio-pharmaceutical chosen.

TECHNIQUE   A. Liver structure scan
Scanning begins approximately 10 minutes after intra-venous injection of the radiopharmaceutical. Multiple views are necessary. The patient is assisted successively into supine, left lateral, left lateral oblique, and prone positions and supported as necessary. A spleen scan may follow immediately and will add 10 to 20 minutes to scanning time.
B. Liver function scan
Rose bengal labeled with ^{131}I is employed in evaluation of liver function since it is metabolized and excreted by the liver in the bile.

The technique is similar to that for liver structure scanning with the following exceptions. Three or four scans may be necessary at intervals determined by the institution. Usually an initial scan is done immediately after injection of the radiopharmaceutical to observe uptake in the liver, a later one to see if the gallbladder has filled, and a final scan after 24 hours.

Usually only anterior and right lateral views are taken during each scan. If it is thought that excretion may be delayed, later scans may be specially scheduled. In some institutions a synthetic fatty meal may be given after the initial scan to stimulate gallbladder contraction.

Lung Scan

PURPOSE

1. Evaluation of pulmonary perfusion by means of a routine lung scan.
2. Demonstration of patterns of air movement and the distribution of air within the lungs by means of a dynamic ventilatory scan.

TIME

1. Rectilinear scanner — 1 1/2 hours.
2. Gamma camera — 30 minutes for a perfusion scan; 5 to 10 minutes for a ventilatory scan.

TECHNIQUE

A. Perfusion lung scan
The radiopharmaceutical is administered intravenously with the patient in a supine position. This is the position of choice when possible, as the influence of gravity ensures the most advantageous distribution of the agent. If the patient is dyspneic and cannot tolerate the supine position, he may be seated throughout the study. When the radiopharmaceutical is a gas in solution, scanning begins 10 to 15 seconds after injection, as perfusion is very rapid. A gamma camera must be used. When a nongaseous agent is employed, scanning begins shortly after injection and four views are usually taken — anterior, posterior, and right and left lateral. A rectilinear scanner may be used in this case, but a gamma camera is preferable since it requires less time. Figure 10-3 compares a typical lung scan with an x-ray.

B. Ventilatory lung scan
The radiopharmaceutical, usually a mixture of xenon 133 and oxygen, is administered by a spirometer. Scanning is begun immediately. It usually involves rebreathing the gas. A mouthpiece is inserted and nose clips are applied for the duration of the test. A gamma camera is used. Figure 10-4 shows the results of dynamic ventilatory scanning.

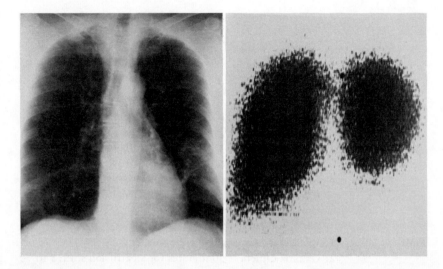

Figure 10-3. X-ray of the lungs (left) compared with perfusion lung scan (right). (Courtesy Philip M. Johnson, M.D., Department of Nuclear Medicine, Columbia-Presbyterian Medical Center, New York.)

PREPARATION 1. A blocking agent may be given depending on the radio-pharmaceutical chosen.
2. The patient should know that:
   a. Deep breathing during administration of the radio-pharmaceutical assists in its even distribution.
   b. More than one scan or type of scan may be necessary to follow the course of his problem and is not necessarily indicative of recurring or increasing ill health.
   c. Any inhaled gas is removed quickly as normal breathing is resumed.
3. If a mouthpiece and nose clips are part of the procedure, the patient should have an opportunity if possible to accustom himself to the feel of the apparatus and to practice breathing deeply with them in place.

PATIENT SENSATIONS The patient may experience anxiety and a feeling of suffocation with the nose clips in place. This feeling may be aggravated if he has a limited respiratory capacity. Assurance must be given that he will be receiving an adequate amount of oxygen through the mouthpiece and will be carefully observed throughout the procedure.

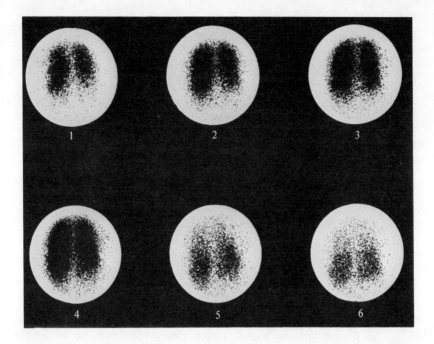

Figure 10-4. Results of dynamic ventilatory scanning using a gamma camera. Images 1 through 4 show the start of inhalation of xenon 133; images 5 and 6 show trapped radioactive particles with patient breathing room air at completion of the scan. (Courtesy Philip M. Johnson, M.D., Department of Nuclear Medicine, Columbia-Presbyterian Medical Center, New York.)

Pancreas Scan

PURPOSE   To evaluate the structure and function of the pancreas.
                 This study is performed primarily for evaluation of pan-
                 creatitis, obstructive jaundice, and cancer of the pancreas.

TIME   1. Rectilinear scanner — 1 1/2 to 2 hours.
                 2. Gamma camera — 20 minutes to 1 hour.

PREPARATION The pancreas has a high degree of affinity for amino acids,
                 which are metabolized by the pancreatic acinar cells into
                 pancreatic enzymes. Therefore the radiopharmaceutical of
                 choice is an amino acid tagged with a radioisotope, usually
                 selenomethionine 75. The aim is maximum stimulation of
                 radioactive tagged pancreatic enzyme production. To achieve
                 this objective some institutions have elaborate preparatory
                 regimens which may include:
                 1. Several days of high-protein meals followed by fasting
                    the night before the scan and a high-protein drink at the
                    time of the procedure.
                 2. Skim milk several hours before the scan.
                 3. Slow intravenous drip of 5% Aminosol (protein hydrolysate
                    injection) during the scan.
                 4. Administration of glutamic acid hydrochloride, propan-
                    theline bromide (Pro-Banthīne), or morphine sulfate at
                    the time of the scan to retard the exit of radioactive
                    enzymes from the pancreas.
                 Some of these preparations may aggravate nausea and an
                 effort should be made to counteract this whenever possible.

TECHNIQUE   A. Rectilinear scanner
                    The radiopharmaceutical is administered intravenously
                    and the patient is placed in a supine position. Foam rubber
                    cushions are used to elevate the left side to a moderately
                    oblique angle. Normally the tail of the pancreas is obscured

by the liver. The object of the oblique position is to cause the liver to fall away from the pancreas, facilitating visualization of the latter. Since the liver also picks up the radiopharmaceutical, the position helps to avoid interfering radiation emissions from the liver. Such interference might increase the difficulty of interpreting the scan. The more obese the patient, the greater will be the degree of obliquity necessary. If the patient is small and thin, the supine position may be sufficient.

The scanner must also be specially positioned to receive maximum radiation emissions from the pancreas. Sometimes a lead shield is placed over the liver to assist in isolating pancreatic radioactivity.

The scan is begun approximately 10 to 15 minutes after injection. Anterior and posterior views are taken, each requiring 30 to 40 minutes.

B. Gamma camera

Scanning begins immediately after intravenous injection of the radiopharmaceutical. Positioning is as for rectilinear scanning, but is accomplished before injection. Since the camera can be adjusted at various angles, screening out of radiation from other organs is simplified. A scintiphotograph is taken immediately after injection to verify proper positioning. Five minutes later another is taken. The patient is then placed in a prone position and after a 5-minute interval, a third picture is taken. An alternate method is to take serial pictures at specified intervals until peak radiopharmaceutical concentration is reached 30 to 60 minutes after injection. In this case the patient remains in the initial position.

At times the physician may elect to perform a liver scan immediately before or after the pancreas scan to obtain a more accurate selective reading and to determine the presence of liver abnormalities. This will extend the length of the procedure.

AFTERCARE   Measures should be instituted to alleviate any nausea and vomiting which may have been precipitated by either the procedure or the preparation for it.

Placental Scan

PURPOSE   Visualization of the placenta to:
1. Determine the presence of placenta previa.
2. Guide the management of patients with third trimester vaginal bleeding.

TIME   1. Rectilinear scanner — 1 to 1 1/2 hours.
2. Gamma camera — 30 minutes.

PREPARATION 1. The patient should be reassured that the amount of fetal radiation exposure is kept to a minimum by the use of a small dose of the radioisotope, and that the radioisotope collects in the maternal blood pool rather than in the fetus or placenta. It should also be emphasized that the test would not be performed without careful evaluation as to its necessity.
2. Immediately before the scan, the patient is asked to void to ensure that no radioactivity from the bladder (the excretory pathway for the radiopharmaceutical) interferes with a clear placental image.

TECHNIQUE   With the patient in a supine position, the outline of the uterus is determined by the physician, who will also palpate and mark the symphysis pubis and the xiphoid process to delineate the borders of the anterior scan. The radiopharmaceutical is administered intravenously and the scan begun within 2 minutes.

After the anterior view is completed, the patient is positioned on her side with knees drawn up to a comfortable level, abdomen supported by pillows, and arms flexed so that her hands rest alongside her face. The greater trochanter and symphysis pubis are located and marked and lateral scanning proceeds. When a gamma camera is used, the lateral view may not be necessary if sufficient information has been obtained from the anterior scan.

AFTERCARE   If placenta previa is confirmed, care is adapted accordingly.

Renogram

PURPOSE

To evaluate:
1. Renal blood flow.
2. Renal tubular cell secretion.
3. Renal excretion rate.

The study is very useful in diagnosing unilateral renal hypertension.

TIME

Thirty minutes to 1 hour.

EQUIPMENT

Although conventional scanning equipment may be used, renograms are often performed utilizing two small probes, one placed over each kidney (Fig. 10-5). The principle of the probe is the same as that of other scanners, but the image produced is a graph with two curves. Each curve represents the individual kidney's pattern of uptake, processing, and excretion of the radiopharmaceutical.

PREPARATION
1. A blocking agent may be given depending on the radio-pharmaceutical chosen.
2. In some institutions hydration with a specific amount of fluid is a requirement for the study.
3. Immediately prior to the procedure the patient is asked to void.

TECHNIQUE

Correct positioning is the most important factor affecting the accuracy of this procedure. Proper positioning is achieved when each kidney is within the field of view of one of the probes or the camera. Sitting is the most desirable posture as it is more anatomically supportive of gravity-induced drainage from the kidneys. If the patient is unable to sit, he is positioned on his abdomen or back. Since the kidneys are retroperitoneal, the aim is to position the probes or scanner so that the energy emitted by the kidneys is not lost

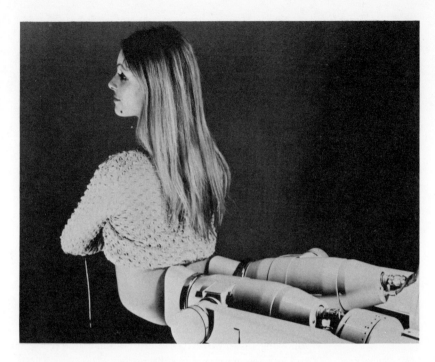

Figure 10-5. Renogram probes in position. (Courtesy Philips Medical Systems, Inc., Shelton, Conn.)

in the intervening abdominal structures before it can be detected. Sometimes a third probe is used to scan the aorta or bladder for comparative radiation values of perfusion and excretion. Should there be any doubt as to the patient's ability to maintain the necessary position, tape may be used to support him. In an additional effort to prevent movement, the scanning device and stretcher or chair are locked into position.

As soon as proper positioning is achieved, the radiopharmaceutical is injected intravenously and the scan is begun. Counts of emission activity are recorded on graph paper every 5 minutes for 1 hour.

Usually a renal scan is done immediately following a renogram unless the patient's condition does not warrant it.

Renal Scan

PURPOSE   To provide information about the gross structure of the kidney and the degree of function of the renal tubular system.

TIME
1. Rectilinear scanner — 30 minutes. There will be a wait of 20 minutes to 24 hours after radiopharmaceutical injection before scanning begins.
2. Gamma camera — 1 hour. There will be a wait of 30 minutes to 2 hours after radiopharmaceutical injection before scanning begins.

PREPARATION
1. If a renogram is also scheduled, it will be done first, as any radiopharmaceutical remaining in the renal cortex following a scan will affect interpretation of the renogram and interfere with accurate diagnosis.
2. The patient is asked to void immediately before the procedure.

TECHNIQUE
1. Regardless of the scanning device chosen, the patient is placed in a prone position.
2. When a rectilinear scanner is used, identifying landmarks may be made on the skin. The kidneys are scanned simultaneously.
3. When a gamma camera is employed, preliminary imaging is done to ensure that both kidneys are in view; if not, they will be scanned separately. Serial images are taken at 2- to 5-minute intervals when the appropriate level of radiation emission is reached.
4. Occasionally a scan may be repeated in 1 to 3 days if results of the initial study are negative.
5. Plain or contrast radiographic studies, or both, are usually performed in conjunction with a scan. Separately, they

may not be conclusive; but when reviewed together, they may yield significant diagnostic information.

6. When a gamma camera is used, a dynamic blood flow study of the kidneys may precede the static scan.

Spleen Scan

PURPOSE To evaluate the structure and function of the spleen.

TIME Ten to 40 minutes.

PREPARATION A blocking agent may be given depending on the radiopharmaceutical chosen.

TECHNIQUE
1. If radioisotope-tagged red blood cells are used as the radiopharmaceutical, a sample of the patient's blood will be drawn prior to the procedure and prepared for injection.
2. Five to 10 minutes after intravenous injection of the radiopharmaceutical, the scan is begun. Three or more views are taken as the patient is successively placed in prone, left lateral, and supine positions.
3. A spleen scan is sometimes combined with a liver scan when it is thought that this will yield additional diagnostic information.
4. Either a rectilinear scanner or a gamma camera may be used.

Thyroid Scan

PURPOSE   To determine the size, position, and function of the thyroid gland.

TIME   Fifteen minutes.

PREPARATION
1. Numerous pharmaceutical agents and other items used in the course of medical management either contain iodine or affect its metabolism in the body, for example, radiopaque contrast media, adrenocorticosteroids, isoniazid, sulfonamides, and radiopaque intravenous catheters. For a complete list refer to the *Physicians' Desk Reference* supplement on nuclear medicine. These items should be avoided in the patient about to undergo a thyroid scan.
2. All jewelry should be removed from the neck and upper chest before the scan begins.
3. The scanner passes laterally across the neck so that it is not always directly over the thyroid gland. The patient should be advised to cough or swallow only when the scanner is to the side. This may necessitate showing the patient the location of his thyroid gland.

TECHNIQUE   The patient is placed in a supine position with the neck hyperextended. The scanner or camera is positioned over the thyroid, and the scan is begun. If a rectilinear scanner is used, its clicking noise increases noticeably as it passes directly over the thyroid gland.

When the study is completed, a physician examines the thyroid gland to correlate any palpable nodules with the information provided by the scan.

PATIENT SENSATIONS   Hyperextension of the neck for the scan may cause the patient to feel as if he were choking. He should inform the technician if this sensation occurs, so that his position may be modified to one of greater comfort.

Bibliography

Early, P. J., Razzak, M. A., and Sodee, D. B. *Textbook of Nuclear Medicine Technology.* St. Louis: Mosby, 1969.

Freedman, G. S. Radionuclide imaging of the injured patient. *Radiol. Clin. North Am.* 11:461, 1973.

Freeman, L. M., and Johnson, P. M. *Clinical Scintillation Scanning.* New York: Harper & Row, 1969.

Gorten, R. J. Nuclear medicine procedures in obstetrics and gynecology. *Radiol. Clin. North Am.* 12:147, 1974.

Johnson, P. C. Benefits and risks in nuclear medicine. *Am. J. Public Health* 62:1568, 1972.

Johnson, P. M., and King, D. L. The placenta evaluation by radionuclides and ultrasound. *Semin. Nucl. Med.* 4:75, 1974.

Kenny, P. J., and Smith, E. M. (Eds.). *Quantitative Organ Visualization in Nuclear Medicine.* Coral Gables, Fla.: University of Miami Press, 1971.

Lorenzo, G. A., and Beal, J. M. Recent diagnostic advances in obstructive jaundice. *Surg. Clin. North Am.* 51:211, 1971.

Maynard, C. D. *Clinical Nuclear Medicine.* Philadelphia: Lea & Febiger, 1969.

Numerof, P. Radioisotopes in liver and pancreatic disease. *Radiol. Clin. North Am.* 8:115, 1970.

Powsner, E. R., and Raeside, D. E. *Diagnostic Nuclear Medicine.* New York: Grune & Stratton, 1971.

Siber, F. J., and Williams, R. C. The use of radionuclides for demonstration of pancreatic and hepatic abnormalities. *Radiol. Clin. North Am.* 8:99, 1970.

Silver, S. *Radioactive Nuclides in Medicine and Biology* (3d ed.). Philadelphia: Lea & Febiger, 1968.

Wagner, H. N., Jr. *Principles of Nuclear Scanning.* Philadelphia: Saunders, 1968.

11

Additional Procedures

Bone Marrow Aspiration

PURPOSE   Aspiration of bone marrow through a needle for microscopical examination.

If an adequate specimen cannot be obtained by aspiration, biopsy is required, using a different kind of needle but a similar technique. Improved needle design has so greatly increased the rate of successful aspirations that this is rarely necessary.

TIME   Five minutes.

LOCATION   Treatment room, physician's office, or patient's bedside.

PERSONNEL   Hematologist and assistant.

EQUIPMENT   A specialized needle, clean specimen slides, and fixative agent. Several types of needle are available, and the choice is up to the physician performing the procedure.

PREPARATION None.

TECHNIQUE   Various sites may be used to obtain a specimen of bone marrow, the most common being the iliac crests and upper portion of the sternum, though the ribs and vertebral spinous processes may also be chosen.

Positioning depends on the area to be punctured:

1. When the site is the sternum or the iliac crests, the patient lies flat on his back.
2. When the posterior ilium is used, the position is like that for lumbar puncture (see pages 15–16).
3. If marrow is to be aspirated from the vertebral spinous processes, the patient sits up and leans forward.

After the chosen area is cleansed with an antiseptic solution, it is infiltrated with a local anesthetic and the specialized needle with stylet is inserted into the bone marrow. The stylet is withdrawn and a 5-ml syringe is attached to the hub of the needle. Manual suction is then applied until bone marrow has entered the syringe. While the assistant prepares slides with the marrow specimen, additional bone marrow is aspirated and placed in a fixative solution. The physician then removes the needle and applies pressure over the puncture site.

PATIENT SENSATIONS

1. A burning sensation is felt while the anesthetic solution is penetrating the skin layers. As the periosteum is infiltrated, the patient experiences a transient sharp pain.
2. When the syringe is held in the position for aspiration the patient experiences pain. Although severe in intensity, it persists for only a few seconds.

AFTERCARE

If the procedure is performed on an outpatient basis, the patient remains in the clinic or physician's office for approximately 30 minutes to ensure that there is no bleeding.

Knee Arthrography

PURPOSE Roentgenographic visualization of the intraarticular surfaces and structures, including the menisci, ligaments, and articulating cartilage.

Most knee arthrograms are performed in an attempt to verify and localize meniscal tears.

TIME Thirty to 60 minutes.

LOCATION Radiology department.

PERSONNEL Radiologist and technician.

EQUIPMENT X-ray table and fluoroscopy unit.

PREPARATION None.

TECHNIQUE
1. The knee is antiseptically cleansed, the adjacent areas covered with sterile towels, and the skin infiltrated with a local anesthetic. The knee joint is entered with a small-gauge needle and any joint effusion is aspirated before the contrast agent or agents are injected.
2. Contrast is attained by injecting into the knee joint a positive liquid agent, a negative gaseous agent, or more frequently both. The injection of both agents creates a double contrast outline of intraarticular structures.
3. The needle is removed and the patient is asked to exercise the joint by walking. If he is unable to walk, the joint is passively exercised by the examiner. This evenly distributes the contrast material throughout the joint.
4. The knee is manipulated under fluoroscopic guidance to position the menisci and other intraarticular structures for optimal visualization. Spot films are taken as the knee is manipulated into various positions.

PATIENT SENSATIONS

1. The sensation of a venipuncture followed by a numb feeling will be felt during infiltration with the local anesthetic.
2. The patient experiences transient pain during injection of the contrast agents owing to distension of the joint.
3. On ambulation the patient may hear a "sloshing" sound caused by the gaseous contrast agent. This will persist for a few days following the examination but in no way interferes with normal activity.
4. Pain may persist after the procedure is completed, and is related to manipulation of the knee.

AFTERCARE

1. The patient is instructed to refrain from strenuous exercise for 12 hours following the examination.
2. Mild analgesics such as aspirin may be prescribed if pain is experienced after completion of the procedure.

Lymphangiography (Lymphography)

PURPOSE   Roentgenographic visualization of lymph channels and nodes to:

1. Determine the extent of lymphomatous disease.
2. Determine the presence or absence of lymph node metastases.
3. Plan portals of entry for radiotherapy.
4. Evaluate lymphedema.

TIME

1. Two hours to prepare for and complete injection of the contrast material.
2. Twenty minutes to expose the appropriate x-ray films.
3. Twenty minutes for a second set of films 24 hours later.

LOCATION   Radiology department or diagnostic suite, or both.

PERSONNEL   Radiologist to inject contrast material; technician to take x-ray films.

EQUIPMENT   X-ray table or reclining chair with elevated footrest similar to a dentist's chair, bright light, mechanical injector for contrast material, and routine overhead x-ray apparatus.

TECHNIQUE

1. With the patient comfortably seated in the specially constructed chair or lying on the x-ray table, the skin on the dorsal surfaces of the feet is scrubbed with an antiseptic solution and the area between the toes infiltrated with a blue dye. The dye is selectively picked up by the lymph system and will identify the lymph channels in the feet within 15 to 30 minutes. The lower extremities are usually studied simultaneously. Upper-extremity and cervical node studies are uncommon, as the findings rarely alter the course of therapy.
2. The skin over an appropriate lymph channel is infiltrated

239

with a local anesthetic and a small incision made. The channel is carefully identified and cannulated with a very small needle joined to a length of tubing. A magnifying glass may be necessary for clear visualization during cannulation. If the lymphatics in one extremity are inaccessible to cannulation, portions of both para-aortic node systems may still be studied, as the contrast material, once it has reached the level of L_3, will be carried by natural lymphatic anastomoses into the other side.

3. The tubing is connected to a syringe containing an oil-base contrast medium. The syringe is in turn fixed to a mechanical device which injects the material at a very slow rate to avoid damage to the small, fragile lymph vessels. Approximately 1 1/2 hours are required to inject 8 to 10 ml of contrast material. If the study is performed on an x-ray table, films may be obtained during the injection of contrast material.

4. Once injection is complete, the needles may be removed, the incision area cleansed and sutured, and sterile dressings applied. However, the radiologist may elect to leave the needles in place until filming is completed. If so, special care is taken to prevent their dislodgement.

5. Preliminary films are exposed to verify filling, followed by a series of films appropriate to the area being studied. Chest films are also taken to evaluate the extent of early oil embolization to the lungs. Normally the oily contrast material passes from the thoracic duct into the venous circulation, lodging in the pulmonary capillary bed. It is eventually eliminated by the reticuloendothelial system. Individuals with normal lungs do not usually suffer any ill effects from this process; in those with borderline pulmonary function the study is contraindicated.

6. Special views are sometimes taken; cinematography may also be used to document dynamic flow. Either of these variations will extend the time required for the study.

7. Twenty-four hours later the patient must return for further x-ray films. These demonstrate lymph node filling. Another chest film is also taken.

PREPARATION   1. Lymphangiography may be performed as an inpatient or outpatient study.

2. The dorsal surfaces of the feet may be shaved and scrubbed with an antiseptic solution prior to the study.
3. Since injection of the contrast material is lengthy and requires remaining immobile, it should be suggested that the patient bring a book, some handwork, or a companion.

PATIENT SENSATIONS

A. During the procedure the patient may experience:
1. The pain incurred by subcutaneous injection of a local anesthetic.
2. Apprehension if allowed to view the surgical exposure and cannulation of the lymph channel.
3. Restlessness during the extended period of contrast medium injection.
4. Some discomfort in the popliteal or inguinal areas at the beginning of contrast medium injection.

B. Following the procedure
1. All patients experience discoloration of urine and stool for 48 hours and a slight soreness at the injection sites.
2. Some patients experience:
   a. Signs and symptoms of significant oil embolization, such as chills, low-grade fever, dyspnea, cough, pleuritic pain, cyanosis, and hypotension.
   b. Mild back or groin pain, weakness, headache, nausea, unpleasant taste sensations, or a combination of these.
   c. Bluish tinge to the skin for approximately 48 hours, and blue discoloration of the feet for up to 1 week.
   d. A slight bluish tinge to the vision for 48 hours.

AFTERCARE

1. The patient should be observed for signs and symptoms of pulmonary emboli.
2. Bed rest is maintained as necessary.
3. The original dressings should remain dry and in place for 2 days following the procedure. Bathing may then be resumed and the dressings replaced by Band-Aids until the sutures have been removed, usually within a week to 10 days.

Bibliography

Angell, F. L. Fluoroscopic technique of double contrast arthrography of the knee. *Radiol. Clin. North Am.* 9:85, 1971.

Dodd, G. D. Lymphography in disease of the liver and pancreas. *Radiol. Clin. North Am.* 8:69, 1970.

Nebe, D. E., and Gavaghan, M. Lymphography and patient reactions. *Am. J. Nurs.* 73:1366, 1973.

Turner, A. F., and Budin, E. Arthrography of the knee. *Radiology* 97:505, 1970.

Wallace, S., and Jing, B. S. Lymphangiography in tumors of the female genital system. *Radiol. Clin. North Am.* 12:79, 1974.

Williams, J. W., Beutler, E., Erslev, A. J., and Rundles, R. W. *Hematology.* New York: McGraw-Hill, 1972.

Wintrobe, M. *Clinical Hematology* (6th ed.). Philadelphia: Lea & Febiger, 1967.

Index